"*The Caregiver's Toolbox* offers an invaluable mix of compassion and information. The authors deeply understand the challenges and trials of caregiving and have created a tools list that kindly helps ease stress and increase competency and organization. This book is an important companion for anyone guiding another through the health care system."

—Deborah Shouse, author of *Love in the Land of Dementia: Finding Hope in the Caregiver's Journey*

"Providing care for a loved one is, for many of us, anything but a simple task. In their superb treatise *The Caregiver's Toolbox*, Carolyn Hartley and Peter Wong outline not only a modern, technology-driven approach to delivering this care, but more importantly, a humanistic one. Exploring how caregivers can leverage such electronic tools as PHRs, physician EHRs, mobile apps, and web portals, the book provides a cost-effective and highly actionable path forward. The authors also expertly walk the reader through many of the financial, legal, and ethical hurdles facing caregivers and do so in a format that is loving, practical, and exceedingly accessible. This is an invaluable resource for anyone who has stepped into the ever challenging yet highly important role of caregiver."

—Robert Tennant, director, Health Information Technology Policy, Medical Group Management Association

"There is an old saying: 'Life is a cruel teacher; first you take the test, and then you learn the lesson.' *The Caregiver's Toolbox* helps simplify and accelerate the process of turning the average person into the extraordinary caregiver. By sharing actual experiences and providing checklists, proven solutions to common problems, and references to other resources, Carolyn and Peter have equipped caregivers to maintain life balance while absorbing the additional demands of providing care to our loved ones."

—Ian K. Gordon, senior vice president, Regence Health Insurance Operations

"My mom is ninety-one and my dad is eighty-nine. I am blessed to have parents that are active, self-sufficient, and in good health. Dad is still managing his rental property business and enjoys the work. Mom loves to be outside and work in her garden. I have thought about it many times but have yet to gather all the information related to my parents' finances and business.

"In *The Caregiver's Toolbox*, Carolyn and Peter lay out a comprehensive road map on how to build a technology plan for your loved one. Their advice on how to start the discussion and how to locate and gain access to financial accounts gives me a starting point to begin the process. The checklists in chapter 4 provide the tools to get organized and make sure all important data is captured. I am finally ready to get started!

"There will be a day when my parents are unable to take care of themselves. Acting now to build a technology plan for my parents will save countless hours and avoid some unpleasant surprises down the road. Thanks to Carolyn and Peter for helping me get started."

—Bruce Honeycutt, chief internal audit and compliance vice president,
Blue Cross Blue Shield of South Carolina

"The authors' suggestion to create a 'Documentation Plan' helped my mother and me prepare for her relocation from a multistory home to retirement patio home living. The Documentation Plan forced us to organize in a thoughtful and complete manner prior to packing up the household belongings. The templates provided in the book helped us purge unnecessary paper, create appropriate electronic back-ups for what was important, and identify knowledge gaps related to infrequently used account information. These practical, easy-to-use tools are a blessing."

—Don Fowler, vice president, client relationships,
Highmark Blue Cross Blue Shield

"As a doctor, I see patients and their families daily who struggle with the challenges of caregiving. Many seem ill equipped for the multifaceted decisions they will face. I have often said that everyone needs a health care advocate, someone within the system who can advise and guide him or her.

"Caregivers often are called on to be the health care, financial, and legal advocates for their loved ones. This responsibility can be a daunting task for caregivers who are unprepared. This masterful book is an essential resource providing a plethora of websites, practical charts, and checklists easily organized so that caregivers are equipped to meet many circumstances.

"During the publishing process, this book had personal application to me and my wife when my uncle and my father-in-law were each referred to hospice. We reread the later chapters, and the information gave us a better understanding and helped us prepare for their deaths. I hope and trust that you and your loved one will derive a great benefit from this remarkable work."

—Randall K. Thomas, OD, MPH, FAAO

"Having been an RN for several years as a director of home health care, having gone through many of these issues you mention with my own father and, now, with a friend who is paralyzed, I think that the content of your book would be so valuable to so many people!

"Caregivers need so much support. Several points I found helpful included the recommendation to express feelings. I found the section on the treasure of walking with someone through the dying process very true in my own experience. I would not trade one single moment of staying with my dad that final month as he died. It is time well invested, and I am so thankful for it. I also appreciated your comments about guilt. I experienced guilt because my dad so wanted to go home, but when it was time for hospice and we had the home alternative, even with my nursing experience, I could not do it. I knew that we needed the support of hospice nurses. It turned out that he did have trouble with secretions, and I was glad he died at hospice. I could ask questions as his loved one, not as a nurse. I even called in the nurse and told her I needed her permission to fall asleep since I feared daddy would die while I was sleeping. She gave me that permission and assured me that many times people wait to die until their loved ones leave the room.

"I also appreciated the section on finding out the wishes of the dying one in terms of plans. A doctor once asked me to serve as a hospice nurse because I love talking with those who are dying about what their wishes are for their memorial service and things like that. I distinctly recall one home health patient whom I gave at-home chemo, and he said his family would not talk to him about his dying, though he felt that he was dying. It was so common and so sad that while his family sat in a separate room watching TV, he shared with me his thoughts about dying. So the tools you are sharing about how to truly help each other as we go through the dying process is so crucial.

"So many of your insights are right on the mark in terms of what caregivers really experience. I pray that the Lord uses your and your coauthor's book to help many people. Thanks so much for sharing with me."

—Tricia Scribner

Also by Carolyn P. Hartley

For Consumers

Working Woman's Communications Survival Guide

How to Be a Master Lobbyist and Still Have Your Mother Love You

For Health Care Professionals

HIPAA Plain & Simple: 1st, 2nd, and 3rd edition

A Guide to Achieving Meaningful Use: Leverage Your EHR to Redesign Workflows and Improve Outcomes

EHR Implementation: A Step-by-Step Guide for the Medical Practice: 1st and 2nd edition

ADA Practical Guide to HIPAA Compliance

Policies and Procedures for the Connected Practice

Technical and Financial Guide to EHR Implementation

Handbook for HIPAA Security Implementation

Field Guide to HIPAA Implementation: 1st and 2nd edition

HIPAA Transactions: A Non-Technical Business Guide for Health Care

HIPAA Privacy for Employers

HIPAA on Demand

HIPAA Privacy for Long Term Care

HIPAA Policies & Procedures Desk Reference

From Patient to Payment: Insurance Procedures for the Medical Office

The

CAREGIVER'S TOOLBOX

*Checklists, Forms,
Resources, Mobile Apps, and
Straight Talk to Help You
Provide Compassionate Care*

Carolyn P. Hartley, MLA, and Peter Wong

TAYLOR TRADE PUBLISHING
Lanham • Boulder • New York • London

Published by Taylor Trade Publishing
An imprint of The Rowman & Littlefield Publishing Group, Inc.
4501 Forbes Boulevard, Suite 200, Lanham, Maryland 20706
www.rowman.com

Unit A, Whitacre Mews, 26-34 Stannary Street, London SE11 4AB, United Kingdom

Distributed by NATIONAL BOOK NETWORK

British Library Cataloguing in Publication Information Available

Library of Congress Cataloging-in-Publication Data
Hartley, Carolyn P.
 The caregiver's toolbox : checklists, forms, resources, mobile apps, and straight talk to help you provide compassionate care / Carolyn P. Hartley and Peter Wong.
   pages cm
 Includes index.
 ISBN 978-1-4930-0802-5 (pbk.) — ISBN 978-1-63076-122-6 (e-book) 1. Medical informatics. 2. Communication in medicine. I. Title.
 R858.H3353 2015
 610.285—dc23

                                        2015009143

∞™ The paper used in this publication meets the minimum requirements of American National Standard for Information Sciences—Permanence of Paper for Printed Library Materials, ANSI/NISO Z39.48-1992.

Printed in the United States of America

To Stan and Eileen. You cared for my sister and my brother with compassion, patience, and sustenance, then held my hand when it was my turn. —CPH

To Mom and Dad, Nancy, Anna, and Daniel. I love you dearly. —PW

Contents

Acknowledgments

For immediately believing in this book, we thank Mary Norris and Jeff Herman, who shepherded this book into your hands. Mary, you turned our passion into a life-altering tool for caregivers and employers who make room for caregivers to be successful employees. Meredith Dias and Bruce Owens, thank you for editorial direction and wisdom. Authors should be so lucky to work with editors as you. Rick Rinehart, you inherited this book and brought it to a new level, for which we are most grateful.

To Stan and Eileen, you taught me how to care with open arms. It is you and the ever-present care you gave to Kathy and Jim that has driven me for the last twelve years to get this book into the hands of our readers.

To Deborah Shouse, my longtime dear friend, former writing partner, family caregiver, and authentic adviser, I thank you for encouragement and your kind words. May your book, *Love in the Land of Dementia* bring continuous joy to caregiving friends.

Thank you, Chris, for enduring my late-night keyboard pecking, back spasms, and continuous requests for a better writing chair. To my daughters, Kristen and Laurie, thank you for your prayers, for your life-giving joy, and for stepping in as my allies in my own caregiving walk. You light the world with the care you offer your children.

To our friends who offer continuous prayer that *The Caregiver's Toolbox* will lighten the load for many, we know you and thank you, especially for the 3 a.m. e-mails. Get some sleep!

I would like to thank Carolyn, my coauthor and coach, whose caring and sharing of her heart encouraged me to write this book with her. What a blessing it is to run the race with you!

Thank you to the friends and clients who shared their stories of struggles, challenges, and tears with me. We acknowledge your request to remain private, but please know your spirit walks with us each day.

Thank you to my sisters, Debbie (Jay) and Susan (EJ), and my brother, Lenny (Gorg), who have shown me each day how to be a caregiver. "How good it is when brothers and sisters dwell together in unity."

Thank you to my wife, Nancy, whose love, patience, and encouragement helped get me through many late nights of writing. You are one in a million! Thank you to Anna and Daniel—I'm so proud to be your dad!

Introduction

Dear, dear Caregiver:

Please accept our highest praise to you for being someone's caregiver. Most likely, you've seen this role heading your way for a while. A recent diagnosis. Aging parents determined to stay in their home. An accident that positioned you as the in-house rehabilitation expert. A beloved child with special needs.

You've talked to family, friends, a spiritual leader for support, gathering resources to help you on this walk. If you are like the 36.5 million other caregivers in the United States right now, you've used up vacation and paid time off, wondering how you will manage time off and duties piling up. If you are among the total 65.7 million Americans who at some time have been caregivers this year, you have a story to tell. Some of your secrets for keeping track of medications, physician appointments, diets, or helping loved ones get in and out of bed or chairs, bathe, or get dressed have made their way into the halls and kitchens of friends and caregiver communities. Thank God for you! Your care contributes more than $572 billion per year in unpaid clinical support. That number is rising because of people living longer (hats off to the Boomers) but fewer people to manage care. Some caregivers tend to more than one person.

If you are like the average caregiver, you spend about twenty-two hours a week providing support. The good news is that in 2014, your weekly devotion topped nineteen hours, one small sign that the aging population may be a bit healthier due to medications, exercise, access to care, long-term care insurance for home-based care, or the rapid expansion of home health agencies.

While love and commitment are at the core of your caregiving, 86 percent of caregivers are untrained, according to a study by the National Alliance for Caregiving. For example, caregivers learn the in-home requirements for managing a patient with Alzheimer's disease or cardiovascular disease. You will learn how to manage the medical bills not only to pay them but also to determine whether they are accurate. You wonder whether your health will be compromised and question whether someone will step in and take over for a while.

My friend, you are not alone. We've been where you are, and we've done it more than once. It wasn't our choice either, but when it was our turn, like you, we stepped up and started making spreadsheets. We've hugged family members so tight that we thought they'd pop; we sat in coffee shops retelling stories that everyone had already heard, but we just weren't done saying what needed to be said. Yes, we held back a few stories that will just have to wait. We got through it with the help of our Lord Jesus Christ, though there were days when we asked the Lord to just cover His ears.

The Caregiver's Toolbox is for list makers, those who wake at 3 a.m. with a list of tasks to do, the ones who remember while unpacking groceries that the prescriptions didn't get picked up. You've bolted way beyond yarn around the finger, and you write reminders in code inside the palm of your hand. Our prayer for you is that you find some peace. Good friends will cry with you when you feel this world is too much. Church or synagogue friends supply meals to carry you through the hardest days or take you out for desperately needed time to breathe.

We prayed for a miracle while we were caregivers, and boy did the miracles happen—joy and such incredible peace from old friends and new ones. We learned the difference between a deep sigh that says "I hurt" and the deep breaths that mean "I love you" or "thank you, my Love." We've cared for those who didn't know that "thank you" could be so difficult to say.

Like you, we were hesitant at first. One thing we had to get over was not to suffer through our role in silence. We learned how to navigate the complex health care system, how to become the advocate when our loved one's voice no longer seemed to resonate with the clinician. We learned how to speak louder when necessary.

We learned to take on health care bills and insurance denials, do background research on billing codes, and ask questions to huffing and puffing billing clerks. We dared to question medications and diagnoses, not that they were wrong or harmful, but we were the frontline care coordinators who built a list of questions when time with physicians eroded to ten-minute pockets of precious access.

We combed through dark closets to find insurance policies and disbursed funds to heirs, trusting that the wills that our beloved family members had entrusted to us would be accurately executed. We became funeral planners and obit writers when God called too many of family home too soon.

As we walked in your shoes, we were sometimes patient, more often not. Sometimes we just needed to slip away, apologize for a gruff tone, and take a five-minute power nap. What we learned is that sometimes our wells were drained by fire hoses; more often than not, our wells were tapped by a steady drip of dos and don'ts. When they ran dry, we found we had little energy to give and that our health hung in the balance. We learned that courage was a liquid substance that on any given day would boil, vaporize, or cool an overheated forehead.

As professionals, we also lost time from work, agonized over customers who needed help faster than we could give it to them. But in every case, neither of us ever bemoaned the time we spent taking care of a loved one. Your story will be different from ours, but the common theme among all caregivers is a giving heart.

We come to you with rich backgrounds in health care. We are major players in the adoption of electronic medical records, complex software that serves as a tool for physicians to track medications, blood sugar, or creatinine levels, and we'll show you some terrific mobile applications available for you. We also have been leading consultants to the nation's top employers and payers, leading work groups to build the electronic medical framework. We've been instrumental in helping health care providers implement privacy and security laws. Be sure to check out our chapter on patient rights.

The Caregiver's Toolbox has your back if you are the early morning list maker. We provide printable checklists you can share with friends who want to know how to help. Here you will find resources and condition-specific communities; you will identify insider tips, resources, patient rights, and health care technology tools.

Technology is disruptive to the old way, but in a good way, it is setting the stage for new innovations. We will continue to post new technology on www.Caregivers-Toolbox.com. Visit us, tell us what you like, and access new apps. Tell us what you'd like to know about or let us know about a cool app that will help others in their caregiving walk.

How to Use *The Caregiver's Toolbox*
The toolbox is divided into three sections based on the stages of a caregiver's time line:

Section 1: Diagnosis
Section 2: Day-to-Day Tools
Section 3: Dealing with Death

You may not go through all of these stages, but begin with the stage that most closely speaks to you and where you may need the most support. You can back up to a previous section, go forward, or hunt and peck through the chapters. If you have purchased this book for a friend or loved one, what a gift you are giving! Your thoughtful gift also means you are committed to helping your caregiving friend through some tough but also joyful times.

It is our hope that you are richly blessed by the tools, stories, and resources provided in this kit. We thought of you every day.

You don't have to be perfect. Thank God, that position has already been filled. You will say things you don't mean, but be strong and wise enough to ask for forgiveness. Please know that we are hugging you through the caregiving process, step-by-step. When you just need a prayer and a friend, send us an e-mail. If it's at midnight, we will answer in the morning, and you'll feel better.

God bless you and your loved ones. We hope you'll let us know how you are doing.

In deepest kindness,
Carolyn and Peter

Section 1

DIAGNOSIS

Caregivers tell us the diagnosis usually signals a first glimpse into what their life might look like for the next three months to twenty years. They also told us the road to being a caregiver is never the same for two people, even within the same family.

This section will help the care partner and loved one work with the medical team to map out a care management program. We start by providing guidance on the three most important events in the diagnostic process, and then we feature mobile or Web technologies that help you navigate through these events:

- Marshall your energy and take in the diagnosis in manageable chunks. Rely on evidence, family, friends, and clergy.

- Get a second opinion. Doctors do, so should you!

- Build your patient and family records. Do it now to help relieve time and paperwork and to coordinate care as you transition from one physician to another.

01 Marshall Your Energy

So now you know. Lab results are in. A pathology report confirmed what you thought may be the case. Or your loved one's accident took more of you than you ever thought would happen. You still have plenty of reasons to expect a happy life, a promotion at work, happy children, and a stable and prosperous career. But right this moment, your life has been tossed into a barrel, and nothing is in focus.

Jessie Gruman, PhD, author of *AfterShock: What to Do When the Doctor Gives You—or Someone You Love—a Devastating Diagnosis*, says, "It's like getting drop kicked into a foreign country without knowing the culture, the language, or a map, but desperate to find a way home." You and your loved ones are confused, flummoxed, and pretty much determined to start fixing things. Who's the best doctor? What hospital will deliver the best outcomes? Build lists of what to do. Hut! Hut! Fix this broken thing.

This chapter is intended to help you manage what some people find to be a crisis. The doctor delivered the diagnosis. Your job now is to corral your knowledge resources and begin building a plan.

In this chapter, we offer a five-step plan to help you answer the most frequently asked question, "What now?" Here you can access the best national and international websites to help develop a plan, find advice from specialists, or connect with others also managing your disease. Many Cool Tools are presented in this chapter, including a self-diagnosis tool to help the patient identify friends, family members, and spouse roles to assist in caregiving.

> When my brother-in-law called to tell me that my sister had been diagnosed with glioblastoma, the most aggressive of brain tumors affecting the central nervous system, I immediately said, "Well let's go after it. I'll get on a flight tomorrow." Reality hadn't quite set in.

I only knew after losing my brother fifteen months earlier to pancreatic cancer that there was something in the family's history—environmental . . . childhood trauma . . . medical? Who cares? We needed to find the one right doctor who knew how to unravel this. I did a mental scan wondering where to jump-start a search for this medical magician. Sloan Kettering? MD Anderson? I'd been working with oncologists in health information technology for years. I knew and had learned to trust many. Time for an all-points bulletin.

"It's terminal, Carolyn."

I was sitting in my office, slowly dropping my head into my hand. The phone grew too heavy for my hand. My sister and I had airline tickets to meet in Minneapolis next month. Even though we lived 1,500 miles apart, we had promised to meet at the Starbucks at the Nicollet Mall every year on my birthday until our minds were too mushy to fly unattended. "Let me make some calls," I said. "I'll find someone who can operate."

Then my brother-in-law, whom I have come to love, respect, and adore as my sister's husband and caretaker, began to weep. I needed to be with him, put my hands on his face, and tell him we could handle this. I could pull off a Mother Teresa healing where the radiation stemming through God's healing mercy would pass through my hand of love, penetrate my sister's brain, and shrink that brain-sucking tumor into a rock so that it could be cut out and pitched like a piece of bad garbage. It was too much. My brother, now my sister. The diagnosis hit me like it was mine to manage. This was my *sister*! My bedroom buddy for fifteen years. I hadn't given her up to be a wife, mother, teacher, skilled horseback rider, and mandolin player just to have her mind blown by some frigging tumor. She was an adored, award-winning teacher, a lover of life. She was sunshine, a school counselor who parented many of the parents in her school district. Even the chief of police sought her advice before sending juveniles to court. I was in shock, and I doubted my brother-in-law could stand up to guide my sister through the health care system.

I was so wrong.

"She has five months, tops. We have a lot of work to do, kiddo."

I had nothing to say, the wind punched out of my stomach.

"You should come when we figure out how we're going to get through this," he said.

Wait? Are you kidding, you want me to wait?

His name is Stan. He is a hero. He became the caregiver who put his life on hold to chauffeur my sister from lab draws to oncologist appointments to radiation and nutrition studies. He helped her into bed, sat with her at the hairdress-ers, and chopped the freshest vegetables into tiny bite-size pieces. Stan also carried with him a spiral notebook so that he could shepherd the details of her lab values, chemotherapy side effects, dosage modifications, and diet restrictions from one provider to another. Moving electronic health information securely from one provider to another was still in its infancy, so Stan became the trusted message carrier between providers. That spiral notebook stayed at their bedside. It was the first and last thing he touched before lying down beside her at night. In an emergency, he could help the emergency room access her medication and chemotherapy regimens so that well-meaning providers wouldn't overdose her. Stan played brain games with her to encourage the few healthy cells to breed new cells. He cleaned up the kitchen when she loaded the dishwasher with liquid dishwashing gel, transforming the kitchen floor into a special effects scene that resembled heaven. He prepared cancer-starving meals and taught her how to swallow nine ginormous chemotherapy drugs a day.

A fellow counselor told him, "You can go into this with your fists clenched and do all the work yourself, or you can open your arms and ask people to help." A private businessman, Stan did what he said he would never be able to do and opened his arms. Friends filled the kitchen with flowers and messages so that, over time, strings of cards wrapped around every window, wall, and doorway in the house.

He created a spreadsheet of tasks asking friends to fill in when he needed to get out of the house for a few hours. Another list tracked foods that my sister should eat and foods to avoid. When others called to see how they could help, he asked them to look at the spreadsheet. If they didn't like any of the tasks, they could add something they wanted to do: take recycling to the street, take his wife for a walk, give the dog a bath, sit with her and make sure she doesn't start the dishwasher.

Each night he raised the bar of how much he loved her and shared the day's experiences with their adult children graduating from medical and state universities. In the rare moments of peace, he researched medical websites and with the help of his daughter the med student searched for clinical trials that might give her a few extra months. None were available for a tumor this big.

Stan was chief financial officer of a midsize organization. Even so, he took a leave of absence to provide full-time care for his wife. His extraordinary em-ployer covered the majority of his salary and told him his position would still be there when he returned.

(Carolyn Hartley)

What to Do When You Receive the Diagnosis

Physicians we've worked with say they prefer to give the diagnosis straight up. They will tell you to take a little time to process the news and then together, working with health care professionals, coordinate a treatment plan. *Take their advice.* While you may experience a diagnosis like this two or three times in your life, doctors see thousands of cases each year. Patients who make the most comebacks are those who take time to think through a strategic plan with friends, with family, and with clergy.

Glenn D. Braunstein, MD, says, "Marshall your energy and resources for a few days. Don't feel pressured into making hasty decisions, especially about significant, invasive procedures or surgery unless you are in imminent danger."

You have plenty of reasons to be confused about how life will change for both you and your loved ones. Shock does that to people. It's the first stage in a caregiver's life. Experienced caregivers tell us that the diagnosis doesn't just happen to the patient. Let's focus on what you will do and what you and your loved one can do together.

Step 1: Research the Diagnosis

The first reaction is to come home and privatize this diagnosis, at least until you can get a handle on it. You may run an Internet search on your diagnosis. Random Internet searches are likely to serve up a combination of both erroneous and trustworthy information, creating even more confusion. Commit to reviewing trusted websites that will give you current symptoms, plain-language descriptions of the diagnosis, and treatment plans.

Put these websites on your search list to learn more about the diagnosis:

- *American Academy of Family Physicians (www.familydoctor.org):* Search for "diseases-conditions."

- *American Medical Association (www.ama-assn.org):* This site provides comprehensive patient information with diagrams and health literacy resources. From the top right side of this website, choose the "Patients" tab. This will direct you to helpful resources.

- *Cedars-Sinai (www.cedars-sinai.edu):* From the blue tabs across the page, choose the "Conditions & Treatments" tab. You can either type the condition into the search field or select the first letter of the condition to find a list of diseases that start with that letter. For example, select "D" if you want to search for "diabetes."

- *Centers for Disease Control (CDC) (www.cdc.gov/DiseasesConditions):* The CDC publishes detailed information about diseases and also provides treatment guidelines as well as public health reporting guidelines.

- *Johns Hopkins (www.hopkinsmedicine.org/healthlibrary/atoz/d):* Johns Hopkins, one of the world's leading medical sources offers a comprehensive library for patients, caregivers and physicians. If you find new information here, print it off and take it to your physician for discussion. Johns Hopkins

Table 1.1. Disease Discovery

Directions: In a quiet place, the soon-to-be-full-time caregiver and patient should begin a discovery process to identify what you know, what you want to know, and how the family can work together to formulate a plan. Begin with what you learned from the doctor. Begin with any educational material you received. Go to websites and search for more information. Make notes on the Disease Discovery form provided here. If it helps, start from the bottom and move up or start in the middle. Anything you write on this page can be changed. For now, you simply are in the discovery stage.

Discovery Questions	Your Answer	What Information Do You Need Now?
What was your doctor's diagnosis?		
What was the first thing you did when you learned of the diagnosis?		
Who can help you make decisions about next steps?		
Have you visited any websites to learn about this disease? What was the URL (Web address?)		
Did your doctor provide you with educational information?		
What members of your family do you want to know about this?		
Is there a time you'd like to tell your family?		
Does your family prefer you blurt it out, or would they want a family meeting?		
Do you want a second opinion?		

and Mayo Clinic collaborate with international hospitals to keep current on new protocols.

■ *Mayo Clinic (www.mayoclinic.org/diseases-conditions):* Mayo Clinic, one of the most world's most frequently researched sites offers details about simple to complex diseases. Physicians frequently access this site for most current treatment updates.

■ *MedlinePlus (www.hlm.nih.gov/medlineplus):* This is a library hosted by the National Institutes of Health that offers a medical dictionary for most diseases and most popular diagnostic searches.

Most disease associations connect patients and families with the basics of the disease. For example, you will find advice on how to live with the disease, survivor stories, and connections to current research on the disease. Some disease categories have competing or collaborating associations. Use your search engine (e.g., Google, Bing, MSN, Netscape, Yahoo!, or Ask) to search for the disease's association. Avoid coming to conclusions, but this is a good time to start taking notes. Use the form in table 1.1 to help guide your research and also help you come back to the same source if you liked the advice. This also serves as an initial response so that you can later return to either see how far you've come or recap your instincts.

Step 2: Contact a Member of the Clergy

Very often, newly diagnosed patients begin to wrestle with how the lives of their family members will change. They also begin looking to God searching for healing, redemption, or answers to raw anger. Friends, family, and the patient are hurting; all need some comfort. This is a good time for you or your loved one to call a pastor, priest, or rabbi and schedule time to talk through your concerns or doubts. During this visit, don't expect your loved one to come to any immediate conclusions but do expect your loved one to question what his or her role should be.

Your loved one may want to go alone. As difficult as it may be, honor that request. A conversation with clergy is very personal. If you are invited to go along, enter the conversation as if you were on holy ground. Be a listener and know that most loved ones are not invited into this sacred meeting. Be at peace with that. Love is not always delivered using words. Hugs are phenomenal healers.

You may want to help your loved one make a list of items to discuss with clergy. As this is a highly emotional time, we provide a list only as a guiding source to help process you and your loved one's emotional and spiritual needs.

"One privilege of ministry is to nurture hope and confront despair," writes Andrew D. Lester in *Hope in Pastoral Care and Counseling.* "When people are wounded and in need of healing . . . hope and despair are major psychological and theolog-

Table 1.2. Things I Want to Discuss with My Pastor (or Priest or Rabbi)

Questions or Discussion Points for Clergy	Key Phrases to Remember from Your Meeting
I've been diagnosed with <name of ailment>, and I don't know how to explain this to my family.	
Why me?	
My family may need help. Who can I call?	
I may need some help as well, but I really am not good at asking for help. Can you give me some guidance?	
Can I maintain some privacy and still have people pray for me?	
Is there a group managing similar diseases in the church who can support me?	
Do you ever coordinate prayer partners?	

ical dynamics." Nearly all newly diagnosed individuals want to know what this disease means and who is there to offer hope.

Use the list in table 1.2 if you need a starting point. A good pastoral counselor will guide you through the meeting. If you are not a member of a faith community, you probably know someone who is. Ask for a referral to the faith leader (pastor, priest, or rabbi). A compassionate listener now will be much more important than a dynamic preacher.

Step 3: Organize Your Thoughts and Build a Tentative Plan

If you are the patient and reading this, you should know that your caregiver and family members are already trying to determine how they can help. Everyone wants this diagnosis to go away and help you return to normal health. That may or may not happen. In either case, you, along with your clinical and caregiving team, will build an action plan, whether it is medication therapy, physical therapy, surgery, professional counseling, radiation therapy, home health, a diet and nutrition plan, or any combination of these. As you and your family continue to explore each chapter, you will learn how to get a second opinion for both the diagnosis and the treatment and how to know whether you should get a second opinion (chapter 2).

As you transition between doctors, hospitals, and care managers, each clinic will ask for the same old paperwork—but we've got Cool Tools for that. In chapter 3, we show you how to standardize your personal medical records in electronic and paper form using the same formats required by physicians who use electronic charting software. The standard format means you don't have to complete all those paper forms every time you see a new doctor.

Because health care is moving into an electronic environment, you will need a technology plan, and you will find guidance on that in chapter 4.

Section 2 helps you transition from discovery into day-to-day caregiving knowledge that helps you lighten your load while empowering you with laws that support you as a caregiver. You will need some technology applications to best use these tools.

Step 4: Explore Mobile Apps to Help

Mobile technology is transforming the way people work, play, and receive medical care. In 2011, more than two-thirds of caregivers were using some form of technology to help them with caregiving, including Web-based calendars, social media, smartphone apps that manage calendar appointments, medication refills, telemedicine visits, and medical hotlines. We provide details about these applications in section 2.

Step 5: Take Care of Yourself

Family caregivers are unpaid family members who have taken on the role of being the primary caretaker of an individual who is ill or unable to manage a disease on his or her own. Care partners may also pay a significant price in lost time, lost wages, fatigue, and failing health.

The average caregiver is a fifty-year-old working female at the peak of her career with an ailing adult living in the home. Most likely, she also has children still living at home. She probably has no formal training on how to take care of the patient/family member but is considering a cut in pay or a transition to part-time work to take on this task. While women, particularly women of color, remain disproportionately likely to take on primary caregiving responsibilities, men have increasingly assumed caretaking duties for children, parents, and relatives with disabilities.

Caregivers also should get a baseline physical exam at the earliest caregiving stages so that you can track your own health. Use this tool to record your vitals. Yes, *you*! Take your vitals to track your own health statistics. You can go to any pharmacy and use the blood pressure cup if you don't have one at home.

It's that last measure, "time for yourself," that seems most lost in the initial phases, but the longer the caregiver provides care, the more essential time for yourself becomes. Every physician, every caregiver book, and every elder care attorney will remind you that you must take care of yourself. Review the list in table 1.4 and check which ones you would like to include in your schedule.

Table 1.3.   Care Partner's Vitals

Vital Statistic	Now	Six Months Later
Blood pressure		
Blood sugar		
Height		
Weight		
Exercise		
Drinking status?		
Exercise		
Smoking status?		
Time out with friends		
Time for yourself		

Table 1.4.   Activity List

Activity	Week 2	Week 3	Week 4	Week 5
Sit in a movie theater, watching comedy while eating warm popcorn laced with Junior Mints. Movies are required, not optional.				
Soak in aromatherapy hot tub with a collection of short stories or novellas.				
Build a blanket fort with chairs like you did as a child and then give your loved one a manicure inside the tent.				
Go on a penny walk. Start walking. Toss a penny. Heads, turn left. Tails, turn right. Might need a compass if you take this too seriously to get you home.				
Create something new through a new hobby (photography, build furniture, paint, learn how to skydive).				
Take up a new sport, one that you can drop and pick up again without having to go through new training.				
Meditate daily and allow God to applaud you. Wait and listen for His warmth to let you know He is there.				

How to Select Your Caregiver

Yes, you do have a choice. You may or may not want to exercise your right to choose. Those of us in a committed relationship have taken an oath: "To have and to hold from this day forward, for better or worse, in *sickness and in health*, for richer or poorer."

The "in sickness and in health" part was a much easier commitment when we were young. An illness then meant taking care of a loved one while recovering from surgery, a bad cold, or a broken bone. These were temporary illnesses. It's much easier to be a compassionate caregiver when the expectation is that the same care will be provided to you when your health is compromised. Long-term illnesses aren't fair. However, illnesses that require caregiving also open doors for deeper levels of communication, love, straight talk, and reconciliation. If you are the patient, highly prize the person (spouse, sister, friend, brother, or parent) who willingly opens him- or herself up to you to assist in your care.

One way to select a caregiver is to ask your physician or a health care professional to help you understand how your disease will stabilize or progress and what your needs will be in the short and the long term. Use table 1.5 to help guide you through your own private chat with yourself. Ask yourself the question, then write the corresponding role (1–5) of the person you believe will provide the help you need. Surprisingly, your answers may not be the same response a family member would offer. Be bold. Would you consider asking your spouse or adult child to also complete this list? Then compare answers.

In table 1.5, read the question, then provide a response as you know it in column 2. In column 3, write the number corresponding with the person most likely to be your primary caregiver:

1 = Spouse
2 = Adult child
3 = In-home nurse or hired aide
4 = Sister or brother
5 = Long-term care facility

Caregiving often is incredibly rewarding, as it slows the hectic pace enough for both patient and caregiver, allowing time together to listen, talk, or share loving thoughts, words, and music or a touch.

Is This Disease in Our Family?

A diagnosis sets off a chain reaction among other family members, making them worry: "Could this disease be in our family?" Family members may hesitate to ask

Table 1.5. Select a Caregiver Questionnaire

Question	Response	Who Can Help with This?
What are the changes my body will make?		
Based on other patients who manage this disease, what is my time line?		
How long will I be mobile?		
Is my mobility dependent on someone lifting me? (Are there devices that can help me get around?)		
Will I be able to make legal decisions about my estate?		
Do I need someone to make legal decisions about my care?		
Can I stay in the home?		
Will I keep my mental capacity?		
How much time each day will be required of a caregiver?		
What services will my insurance policy cover?		
Do I have long-term care insurance? For in-home, skilled nursing facility, or both?		
To whom should I give legal authority? (See also chapter 7.)		
Will I need physical care in the home following treatments?		
Will I need transportation to and from treatment facilities? Does someone need to stay with me during treatment?		
Who will provide my caregiver and me with emotional support?		
Will I need help taking medications?		
Who will track my body's changes for better or for worse? Do I want to know about the changes?		

(continued)

Table 1.5. (*continued*)

Question	Response	Who Can Help with This?
Who will communicate with friends and family about my condition?		
Who will keep visitors away from me when I don't want them in my room?		
Do I have a living will identifying whether to keep me on life support?		
Have I given legal authority to someone who will act on my behalf (e.g., durable power of attorney) if my spouse is no longer living?		
Did you complete this with one or more of your "1–5" team members?		
Total	1 (Spouse) = _____ 2 (Adult child) = _____ 3 (In-home nurse) = _____ 4 (Sibling) = _____ 5 (Skilled nursing) = _____	
What are your next steps?		

about hereditary diseases because it makes them appear to be self-involved rather than compassionate about the diagnosis. The question won't go away and more likely will interfere with the patient–caregiver relationship. Face this one head on. This is a conversation you should have with your own physician. While most health care professionals are not keen on patient self-diagnosis tools, they also recognize that consumers have a right to learn about genomic influences in the family without spending significant amounts of money on lab tests. Share results of lab tests with your physician, who will help relieve or explain unnecessary anxiety.

Cool Tools for Health-Aware Consumers

- Any Lab Test Now helps families with high-deductible insurance get tested for 8,000 non–life-threatening conditions, such as high blood pressure, pregnancy, strep throat, urinary tract infections, and diabetes maintenance panels. Any Lab Test Now then can send results to telemedicine services for a doctor's review and possible prescription.

- Illumina is a cancer-testing platform that runs huge numbers of standardized tests to guide therapy for cancer patients. As of January 2014, this is the only genomic testing service that broke the $1,000 cost barrier. Most states require you first obtain a prescription for genomic testing. Not all physicians are aware of affordable genomic services. We offer Illumina as one possible source.

- Companion Dx is a secure network that disseminates genetic test results with licensed health care professionals, enabling them to optimize the use of drugs likely to be most effective.

About Caregivers

- Approximately 65.6 million people in the United States have served as unpaid caregivers to adults or children outside of normal parenting responsibilities.

- A caregiver may provide support over a long period of time, such as to a family member with complex conditions (e.g., diabetes, Alzheimer's disease, failing eyesight, and hypertension), or over the short term, such as a family member recovering from major surgery or diagnosed with life-threatening or terminal illness.

- In most cases, caregivers are unpaid family members who have taken on the role of being the primary caretaker of an individual who is ill or unable to manage a disease on his or her own.

- The average caregiving lifespan is 4.6 years with one-third providing more than five years of caregiving.

- Eighty-five percent of all caregivers do *not* know how to be a caregiver, and 66 percent of all caregivers are women working full-time. Six out of ten caregivers say that the out-of-pocket costs make it difficult for them to pay for their own basic necessities, and 63 percent say that they are no longer investing for retirement while caring for a loved one.

Table 1.6. Caregiver Profiles

Percentage	Population	Task
29%	All adults in America	Are caregivers
79%	Family caregivers	Provide care to someone over 50 years old
60%	All caregivers	Work full-time
66%	All caregivers	Are women
60%	All caregivers	Make work-related adjustments
10%	All caregivers	Reduce hours to part-time
51%	All caregivers	Are 18 to 49 years of age; average age is 48
21%	All households	Provide care for an ailing member in the home
15%	All households	Drive more than one hour to care for someone
85%	All caregivers	Do *not* know how to be a caregiver
38%	All caregivers	Look to the Internet for advice

Source: National Alliance for Caregiving.

■ According to a study by Evercare, commissioned by UnitedHealthcare and the National Alliance for Caregiving, family caregivers who are the backbone of our health care system represent an economic value of $375 billion to the nation's economy for the care they deliver to loved ones.

Key Takeaways

In this chapter, you learned the following:

■ Find trusted medical websites to help you get a better sense of the diagnosis

■ Build your caregiver network and identify educational resources

■ How to marshall your energy to develop a plan for your new approach to living

■ How to track your own vitals to measure your own quality of life

Somewhere in the discovery process, you may have thought this doesn't feel right; the treatment plan isn't aggressive enough, or it's too intense. You want a second opinion. If a second opinion is on your mind, chapter 2 directs you to the right resources. In chapter 2, you will learn how to ask your doctor for a second opinion without feeling guilty. You'll learn what to expect and who pays for this opinion.

Do You Need a Second Opinion?

Second opinions can save lives. Health care professionals seek second, third, fourth, and fifth opinions and then consult national experts. You should consider doing the same without feeling a drop of regret.

In this chapter, we provide guidance on the following:

- What a second opinion is.

- How to ask for one without being confrontational or without jeopardizing your physician–patient relationship.

- How to obtain a second opinion so that it brings real value to you and your loved one. You may find that a second opinion also opens the doors for innovative surgeries, clinical trials, or more aggressive or alternative treatment.

- How to manage costs for a second opinion.

- How to search for a physician's clinical success rate.

- How to find the hospital's history of delivering quality care to keep you safe and infection free during your stay.

- If you decide that the best care is in another country, we will provide you with guidance on what to look for, how to know whether you will be safe, where to stay, and how to plan for the trip.

If you don't believe a second opinion on a diagnosis or treatment plan is right for you, then move on to chapter 3, where you will learn more about how to securely build your patient and family medical records.

What to Expect from a Second Opinion

In seeking a second opinion, most likely you seek guidance to achieve any of the following:

- Confirm the diagnosis.

- Evaluate the prescribed treatment plan, surgery, or procedure.

- Consider an alternative treatment plan.

- Evaluate whether the lab results have changed or been misread.

A second opinion should come from a licensed clinical professional who has been practicing in your diagnosed disease area for at least five years. This may be an internal medicine physician, a specialist, a national clinic that influences disease treatment plans, or a medical professor at an academic medical center. An Internet search is not a second opinion. However, an Internet search may be a good place to learn more about your disease category and find a specialist.

A second opinion may be required by your insurance carrier prior to performing higher-risk procedures. For example, many insurance companies, including Medicare, are likely to require a second opinion. Elizabeth Cohen's story on CNN Medical News reported on the "Five Diagnoses That Call for a Second Opinion":

- A procedure that comes with a risk of dying, stroke, or severe infection

- Hysterectomy

- Pregnancy termination for fetal abnormality

- Treatments for brain tumors

- Treatment for varicose veins when evidence indicates it may be deep-vein thrombosis or a blockage

As a means to empower you or your loved one to seek a second opinion, first take a look at how your doctor is most likely to determine a diagnosis and develop a treatment plan. With this knowledge, you can build a case for seeking additional medical counsel.

Second opinions can cause you to slip into a loop of indecisive action, leaving you without a definitive plan to care for yourself or your loved ones. To prevent this, set a deadline that limits the amount of time you will spend searching for additional clinical advice and focus on treatment.

How Doctors Determine a Diagnosis

Doctors are scientists looking for evidence to help better understand why you have come into the medical office (your reason for the visit, or a "problem list"). They are trained in medical schools to very quickly take in volumes of data, such as your age, gender, occupation, race, marital status, vitals, current medications, allergies, habits such as smoking and alcohol use, skin color, blood pressure, temperature, height, and weight, all within about ninety seconds. Information comes to them in subjective and objective processes:

> *Subjective:* Subjective experiences are influenced by your opinions, interpretations, and past experiences. Your physician often begins a visit by asking, "How do you feel," to learn more about your reason for the visit. Events in your life, such as a relative moving in with you or a new pet, influence your health and treatment outcomes. An attentive physician will want to know about those as well.
>
> *Objective:* Consider the root word "object" to help you remember the difference between objective and subjective. An object is something you can touch and feel. When analyzing objective data, your physician takes in hard facts and scientific evidence that can be verified. For example, the nurse may use a blood pressure cuff and take your blood pressure two times: the first to get rid of cuff anxiety and the second to get a balanced reading. A nurse treating a patient with heart disease is likely to check blood pressure in both arms to determine if the heart is pumping blood evenly.

The amazing part of the physician's training is the ability to also put aside any personal events going on in his or her life and to dismiss findings from the last person who was examined to focus completely on you. Prior to coming into your exam room, the nursing staff entered details from your "intake exam" into the computer and also likely had a side conversation with your physician to indicate how you or your loved one is holding up. This clinical evaluation process works very well for your clinical team so that the doctor is prepared to greet you.

Chronic illnesses, diseases that build or worsen over a period of months or years, often create a mix of objective data. One reason is that if you are managing a chronic illness, you also may be battling a combination of multiple diseases, such as heart disease, arthritis, and cancer. The doctor is likely to order tests or procedures to help sift through the variables and confirm or alter the physician's suspicion about the diseases' progress.

Assessment

A diagnosis for a complex chronic illness usually begins with a thorough physical examination of your body's systems, your vitals, medications, and allergic reactions to prescriptions and over-the-counter drugs you have taken. The examination also includes a review of medical and surgical history, your family's medical history, your smoking and alcohol habits, exercise routines, and work environment to reach a clinical decision about what may be causing your chronic illness to degrade or improve.

Sometimes test results are inconclusive. The doctor may then request even more laboratory tests or procedures to better understand what's going on inside your body. Additional tests may include an X-ray, a PET (positron-emission tomography) scan, a sonogram or mammogram, blood or urine tests, a tissue sample, or a biopsy. Your doctor may also have requested magnetic resonance imaging (MRI), which takes pictures of organs and structures inside the body. You may wonder why it took the doctor more than one visit to finally order an MRI when you thought one should have been ordered in the first place. The reasons include the following:

- Your insurance company or payer requires multiple diagnostic procedures before authorizing an MRI or a PET scan, as they not only are costly but may be unnecessary as well.

- The practice load may be backed up or short staffed today, and there isn't enough time to focus deeply on you. For example, Mondays and Fridays are usually very busy days.

- A scientific disease organization has published findings, or *clinical protocols*, that suggest the physician should request more tests.

Plan

Until now, the physician has completed the subjective, objective, assessment portions of your visit and now establishes a plan. Notice that the initials for these words spell the word SOAP, a commonly used acronym in clinical decision making. Your treatment plan is usually guided by clinical protocols.

Clinical protocols developed by disease management clinical associations, such as the American College of Obstetricians and Gynecologists (women's health) or the American College of Cardiology (heart health), help determine appropriate treatments for diseases diagnosed by the physician. A protocol is scientifically based medical evidence that the treatment or combination of tests and procedures will produce a reliable outcome. If the physician does not follow clinical protocols and his or her independent treatment plan results in a medical error that is damaging to you, he or she may need to explain to a legal team or a medical review board why he or she decided not to follow protocol. Protocols may be challenged and altered, but new treatment guidelines generally happen as a result of a comprehensive clinical studies.

New protocols (or treatment guidelines) also would not emerge if it weren't for physicians and scientists taking a chance that there is a better way to treat or cure your disease. New surgical techniques and chemotherapy regimens (a combination of drugs and the amount and the length of time the drug is injected) come as a result of doctors scientifically experimenting with new approaches in order to save or improve the quality of life for patients. Doctors go to international medical meetings to learn more about new medications or innovative surgical procedures that have not yet been approved by the U.S. Food and Drug Administration. But not all doctors can get away from daily patient care to attend medical meetings in Germany, Belgium, Norway, Turkey, or Israel, so many of them learn about innovative treatment through online and medical society courses.

The point here is that there may be research, studies, innovative treatment plans, or drug research conducted in another part of the country or of the world that your doctor doesn't know about or hasn't taken into account. That's why medical professionals seek second opinions and why we suggest you do the same.

How to Ask for a Second Opinion

Most likely, you trust your doctor, or you would have found another more to your liking long before you needed a caregiver. As a result, it may not feel natural to ask for a second opinion, fearing you will offend the clinical staff. If you are concerned about offending your doctor, bring along a family member who will serve as your advocate.

Here are a few approaches you can use when asking for a second opinion:

Family approach: "Dr. Smith, Our family has a lot of decisions to make about my care, and one of the things I promised them is that I could get a second opinion about how best to proceed. Is there a specialist that you recommend I consult?"

Own it: "Dr. Smith, I've been doing a lot of research on this disease, and I'd like to get a second opinion before we proceed with this plan. Is there a specialist that you recommend I consult?"

Blame-the-spouse approach: "Dr. Smith, my wife will hang me out to dry if I don't get a second opinion. Who is the nation's medical super star I can talk to?"

Keep it to yourself: Thank the doctor, pay your bill, and call a friend for advice. Before you leave, though, you must have a plan: follow the investigative approach first.

Investigative approach: Patients are poor health care investigators, but they are great investigators when it comes to retail shopping. To be a good comparison shopper, you must have some preliminary details. If you are purchasing a dress, you want to know your dress size. If tires are on your mind, you need to know your car's wheel size and typical weather or terrain hazards before making a purchase.

The same is true for health care. You cannot be a comparison shopper if you don't know what to compare. Use the list in table 2.1 to get started.

In health care, doctors are quite willing to provide you with a summary of your lab tests, MRI results, suspected diagnosis, pathology results, and much more. If they forget, just ask. If you are feeling shy about asking for these documents, know that the Health Insurance Portability and Accountability Act of 1996 (HIPAA) entitles you by law to receive each item mentioned in this checklist. (We discuss HIPAA and your rights in chapter 8.) You may need to sign permission forms to obtain additional information from prior visits, but the paperwork is there only to help define what you need from your chart. Use the checklist in table 2.1 to help you build a file for your second opinion and also for your personal medical records.

Table 2.1. Documents to Collect from Your Physician's Practice

What to Ask For	Why You Need It	Did You Get it?	
		Yes	No, Because . . .
Test results	You want a plain-language interpretation of <lab>, <sonogram>, <pathologist> test results. Not all doctors can generate a plain-language description from their electronic medical chart, but the doctor or nurse is required by law to be sure you understand what the lab results mean to you. If a biopsy report indicated cancer, you want to know the tumor size, the number of tumors, and what stage you are in (stage I, II, III, or IV).[1] Staging also helps doctors determine how to treat the site of the original tumor.		
The physician's treatment plan	A treatment plan describes how the physician plans to treat your illness or disease. This includes any single step or a combination of next steps, such as a prescription with a follow-up visit,		

1. Tumor staging is the process of finding out much cancer is in the body and where it is located. For more information about tumor staging, go to www.cancer.org/treatment/understandingyourdiagnosis/staging.

What to Ask For	Why You Need It	Did You Get it?	
		Yes	No, Because . . .
	surgery, radiation, a chemotherapy plan, diet and a nutrition plan, a referral to another doctor, more tests, or a combination of these and other recommendations. A family member is a great ally for asking the hard questions and taking notes if you aren't sure about the treatment plan. You don't have to agree to the plan, but you should listen and take notes. In a patient-centered medical center, a case manager or nurse will follow up with you to ask how well the treatment plan is working for you and advise you or your caregiver on home activities.		
A clinical summary of your visit	A clinical summary is a recap of your visit and includes the following: • The doctor's contact information • Things you should do after the visit • Tests the doctor ordered • Patient instructions • An updated medication list • Updated vitals • Your reason for today's visit • Any updates to your current problems • Immunizations or medications administered during the visit • A summary of topics covered • Your next appointment • Scheduled tests, if scheduled while you were there The clinical summary (also called patient summary or after visit summary) provides recommended decision aids to help you take charge of your health. Most electronic health record systems can produce a clinical summary for each visit.		

(*continued*)

Table 2.1. (*continued*)

What to Ask For	Why You Need It	Did You Get it?	
		Yes	No, Because . . .
	Your doctor may tell you the practice will download your chart into a patient portal within one to two days following your visit. You can access your clinical summary using your own user ID and password.		
Educational material about your disease	Your physician or nurse should either print or hand to you educational material about your disease, including how you can manage your disease at home. Whether you seek a second opinion or not, you should receive this.		
Your doctor's name	Write down the doctor's name, his or her nurse's name, office phone and fax numbers, and the name of any clinical person involved in your visit. You may need this for your second opinion.		
Superbill	A superbill is a sheet of paper with charges and codes that define your services and how much you paid out of pocket. This may be printed in triplicate or printed from the computer. If on paper, the doctor or nurse hands the superbill to you as you are walking out of the exam room. The doctor tells you to give this to the person at checkout, who separates the three pages and hands you the pink or yellow copy. Your superbill also may be electronically printed and serves as your receipt for payment. Most people throw this away. *Do not* throw this away.		
	Your superbill also contains a list of codes used to define the reason for visit (why you are sick). There are all kinds of hidden codes on this page that we will discuss in chapter 7.		

What to Ask For	Why You Need It	Did You Get it?	
		Yes	No, Because . . .
Current medications	Embedded in the electronic chart is a list of active medications that all licensed physicians have ordered for you and that your insurance company has paid for from your pharmacy benefits plan. Only a licensed clinician may access this list to ensure they don't prescribe a medication that creates a dangerous reaction with one you already take. You want to check this list to be sure it is accurate.		

How to Find Your Second Opinion

Ideally, the physician you want to consult is a specialist in your disease category. A second opinion is not an indictment against your current physician, but you have an obligation to yourself and your family to find a doctor who has conducted innovative research or is setting new clinical protocols that have not yet been adopted specialty-wide.

There are a few ways to find your potential medical superstar:

1. *Science Daily*, a consumer publication that highlights innovative medical research, including new medical procedures. A few articles that may be of immediate interest to you are these:
    a. "Robotic Surgery for Pancreatic Cancers." This article offers innovative surgical processes for surgically removing pancreatic cancers without removing parts of your stomach, spleen, kidneys, and pancreas.
    b. "Stress Urinary Incontinence: Minimally Invasive Operations As Effective As Open Surgery."
    c. "Emerging Stem Cell Treatments." Used in other countries for decades, stem cell treatments offer exciting possibilities, but you may need to go to another country to receive certain stem cell therapies.
2. Conduct a literature review on your diagnosis. Doctors looking for answers to medical problems like yours publish their findings from observational studies. Let's go find them. Here's how to do that:
    a. Log on to your Internet search engine.

b. Type in the name of your disease and then add one of the following key words:

    i. *British Medical Journal (BMJ): BMJ* publishes studies from around the world but especially from European countries.

    ii. *Journal of the American Medical Association (JAMA).*

    iii. *New England Journal of Medicine (NEJM).*

    iv. *National Institutes of Health (NIH).*

c. You don't have to understand all the clinical details in the article, as most are written in scientific and medical terms. Read the abstract. This is the article's executive summary. See if the study findings apply to your disease.

d. Look for the name of a physician or physician group that authored the article. Usually the first author is the lead researcher, and the last name is the professor assigned to oversee the study. You want the MD, but you may also want to contact the professor (last name) to learn why he or she supported the study. As a rule, doctors who publish are in high demand, meaning that they are the go-to person for physician referrals.

e. Look to see how many participants are in this doctor's study. If this is a surgeon demonstrating a new surgical technique, you want evidence that he or she has conducted 500 to 1,000 successful surgeries.

f. You may have a difficult time getting an appointment with recently published doctors, but there are ways to manage this as well:

    i. Ask your physician to open the door for you by referring you to this specialist.

    ii. Find out where this doctor practices and read his or her bio posted on the website.

    iii. Call the practice and tell the person who answers that you were reading an article in the <name of journal>, and you'd like to learn more about his or her availability to see you. Remember, doctors publish so that other physicians (and patients) will find them.

    iv. You may have a friend or family member who has heard of this person. If so, leverage the relationship. "I've been referred to you by one of your former patients, <name of patient>. Don't make up this person. With a few simple mouse clicks, the practice can verify your friend's name.

    v. If the practice says the doctor is not taking new patients, ask who in the practice works with the doctor and ask for an appointment with the published doctor's colleague.

3. Reached out to world-renowned physicians through online or telemedicine appointments:

    a. MyConsult Online is a medical service offered by Cleveland Clinic. It takes about forty-five minutes to complete the documentation, and you will need your medical record. (Pull together content from table 2.1.) This service may be sponsored by your employer, but if it is not, be sure you have approximately $500 to $750 available on your credit card or ask your insurance plan if they will cover the cost of this consult. Most health insurance plans do not cover online second opinions at this time, but it doesn't hurt to ask. You also will need the diagnosis provided by your physician. You can find this on the bill you received when leaving the physician's office. You also likely received educational material on this diagnosis before leaving the practice. MyConsult will also request results of studies, such as lab tests, MRIs, and symptoms. You can print off this list and use it as a reference tool.

    b. Johns Hopkins Medicine also offers remote medical second opinions, and the cost is about the same as Cleveland Clinic. There may be additional costs in any online second opinion for additional pathology or radiology interpretations.

    c. Online second opinions cannot be used instead of an initial in-person visit. The physician completing the second opinion must access information you received from your primary care physician or specialist.

Conduct Background Research on the Specialist and Treatment Facility

Most patients and families immediately turn to the Internet to learn more about their physician or hospital. For example, if you searched for your physician on Google or Bing, the results would direct you to Healthgrades.com, Vitals.com, Yelp.com, Ratemds.com, or UCompareHealthcare.com. These are free services with advertising-supported websites. These ratings do not determine the physician's clinical capabilities; rather, these sites report on how well the patient believes he or she was treated.

Physicians generally appreciate patients who look for personal reviews on how well they manage and respond to patient needs. To help with ratings, some purchase services to help boost or manage their ratings. From a business perspective, that's good marketing because most services also report to the practice patients who had an unsatisfactory experience. This allows the practice time to improve quality care and repair the relationship.

You also can search for a physician by looking first to hospital ratings. Hospitals are very competitive and have the resources to report whether they are meeting quality benchmarks somewhat easier than physician practices. Hospitals also generally employ quality control officers who gather information about the patient's treatment, how well the patient responded to care, the length of time a patient stays in the hospital, and any reportable patient safety event.

Our favorite websites for evaluating hospital ratings are these:

1. US News and World Report, *US News Best Hospitals:* Rankings are collected yearly in July and combine data from patient satisfaction, death rates, patient safety events, and physician ratings on hospitals they consider the best in their specialty for difficult cases. *US News* collects data for sixteen specialties.

   Begin your search by selecting one of the sixteen disease areas, from cancer to urology. For example, select "Cardiology and Heart Surgery." While at this website, you will find a national rank of clinics and their scores. We recommend you select a hospital or two near you to view their Scorecard and location. Say you select "Cleveland Clinic." You can either scroll down to view this clinic's adult specialties or select from the Overview the following menu: "Rankings, Patient Satisfaction, Stats & Services or Doctors." *US News* does not rate doctors, so a search for one specific doctor can be frustrating.

2. *Consumer Reports Hospital Safety Analysis:* You will need a subscription to *Consumer Reports* to access the complete study, but the report compiles data on how many people were readmitted to the hospital within thirty days of discharge; overuse of CT scans, which can cause cancer many years later; hospital-acquired infections; how many patients had a heart attack, heart failure, or pneumonia and died within thirty days of entering the hospital; and the number of treatable but fatal complications after an operation.

3. *Medicare Hospital Compare:* If you use this website, be sure to check out the American College of Surgeons voluntary reporting on what happens to patients after three types of surgery: lower extremity bypass restoring blood flow to the lower leg and foot, colon surgical outcomes, and outcomes for patients sixty-five years of age or older. The American College of Cardiology also voluntarily participates by reporting how many patients are readmitted to a hospital after a percutaneous coronary intervention, which is a process to open blocked blood vessels that can cause a heart attack.

How Much Will My Second Opinion Cost?

Earlier, we presented online second-opinion services. But many patients prefer an in-person second opinion from a specialist in your geographic area. You can best manage the cost by being prepared and bringing with you a comprehensive medical record (see table 2.1) you obtained from the physician who initially diagnosed your condition.

Before scheduling a consultation with the specialist, call your insurance company and tell them you have some questions about a recent diagnosis (or treatment plan) and would like to schedule a second opinion with <name of physician>. Your insurance company will tell you whether this specialist is in network or out of network, what your benefits package will pay, and your copay. To make this call, you will need the following:

- Your health insurance card

- The subscriber's name and the last four digits of the subscriber's Social Security number

- A phone number where you can be reached

If your insurance benefits plan does not cover the costs of a second opinion, don't hang up but *do* ask the following questions:

- If I pay out of pocket for this visit, what would be the allowable amount that you would have reimbursed the specialist? In general, the allowable amount is 35 to 75 percent of the physician's bill. (We discuss how this happens in chapter 7.)

- If I pay out of pocket for this visit, who should I talk to at the practice to get a reduced bill?

Depending on the advice you receive from your insurance company, call the practice to schedule a consultation with the specialist. By now, you will have general knowledge of your financial responsibilities. A consultation is typically twenty to thirty minutes but may be extended, depending on your situation. When scheduling the consult, ask these questions:

- How much does <doctor's last name> charge for a consultation?

- What is your practice's fee if I pay out of pocket?

If the answers are the same, it's time to call the practice's billing department and negotiate an out-of-pocket fee, especially if you suspect that your health insurance plan will not cover this consultation. If this is a small practice, ask to speak with the practice's office manager. Your conversation will go something like this:

- I plan to pay for the specialist's consult out of pocket. What are his or her fees to me?

- Can I get prebilled, or would you send me something before the appointment so that I know how much to bring? (Your prebill will serve as evidence for your payment for a consultation in the event you believe you are being charged more than agreed on.)

If you and the specialist agree to proceed with treatment following the consultation, you *and* the specialist's practice should circle back with your insurance company to be sure the next steps will be authorized for payment.

What to Bring with You on Your Second-Opinion In-Person Visit

You've gathered information from your second-opinion work plan, and now it's time to pull this together into a file. Use table 2.2 to provide information for your in-person visit.

Table 2.2.   What to Bring on Your Second Visit

What You Need	Where to Get It	Do You Have It?
Your insurance card	Your insurance company will provide this.	
Your driver's license or photo ID	Probably your wallet.	
Preauthorization certification	Your insurance company may or may not pay for this visit. Call the number on the back of your insurance card and verify your out-of-pocket costs. If you receive a preauthorization, bring it with you.	
Name and location of the practice	Your second opinion may be at an academic institution, making it somewhat difficult to navigate through the campus. Bring a detailed map that also describes available parking places.	

What You Need	Where to Get It	Do You Have It?
Hospital where the physician is affiliated	Many published physicians are affiliated with an academic medical center. Learn about the hospital's rankings through several sources: *US News & World Report* or Medicare.gov.	
Local hotels	If you are traveling long distance to see this physician, find the name of nearby hotels. Often the hospital's website provides the name and location of hotels, ratings, and distance to the hospital.	
Medication list This includes a list of all current prescribed and over-the-counter medications, dosages, and how you take them (orally, by injection, or topically).	These may be in your medicine cabinet, under-the-sink baskets, vitamins, over-the-counter drugs, and painkillers. Read the label to access dosage amounts.	
Allergies	Your allergies should include allergies to any medication, food allergies, or airborne allergies (pollen).	
Surgical history	Most physicians want a list of surgeries you've had in the past ten years, but others may want to go back twenty to thirty years. You can learn how to build this history in chapter 3.	
Family medical history	Bring the family history chart from chapter 3. This is especially important to help the physician analyze possible genetic, environmental, cultural, or work-related diseases.	

(*continued*)

Table 2.2. (*continued*)

What You Need	Where to Get It	Do You Have It?
Lab results	Bring all lab results that you believe may be relevant.	
Clinical summaries	This is the clinical summary from your physician's patient portal. If you see multiple physicians and have multiple patient portals to access, you should create your own single source. Learn more in chapter 3.	·
Diagnosis	The diagnosis can be found on your superbill. It also is on the clinical summary.	
X-rays and diagnostic imaging tests, such as MRI, CAT or PET, and DXA scans	Your second-opinion specialist wants the original X-ray or CD that contains your MRI. Call the hospital or clinic and get a copy of the actual film or CD. There may be a small charge to obtain this, but there will be a much larger charge if you have to pay for another MRI.	
Narrative report of findings from your X-rays or MRI	The second-opinion specialists may agree or disagree with the original narrative report but may also want to read it. This report is not a visual representation but, rather, a professional clinical interpretation of your images.	

What If Your Second Opinion or Advanced Care Is in Another Country or Another State?

If you seek care from a physician in another state, first check to see if the physician is "in network" with your insurance payer. The physician also may have a reciprocal billing agreement with your practice. Always check with your health insurance company first. Out-of-country second opinions follow a different process.

In March 2014, *Science Daily* featured a story about minimally invasive (little to no cutting) brain surgery developed in Israel and tested at Johns Hopkins Hospital. In testing, doctors at Johns Hopkins found that the brain surgery more accurately identified the source of disease and streamlined the surgical process with improved patient safety outcomes using equipment already common in the operating room.

Thailand boasts that its Western-trained physicians and surgeons have helped Bangkok Hospital become one of the largest hospitals in the world, treating patients along the spectrum from cosmetic surgery to heart bypass surgery. In 2005, the hospital treated 150,000 medical tourists, and by 2015, the hospital expects to earn $3.22 billion from patients and family members, blending a family vacation with a medical procedure. Bangkok, Chiang Mai, Hua Hin, Koh Samuim Pattaya/Chonburi, and Phunket are some of the more recent destinations that lure patients from the United Kingdom, the United States, the Middle East, Germany, Australia, and Japan.

The earliest adopters of medical tourism stemmed from in vitro fertilization clinics in destinations such as Buenos Aires, Costa Rica, and Thailand. The treatment combines a relaxing trip with American and Western-trained gynecologists who have expanded their services into less regulated destinations, resulting in a higher number of live births.

Istanbul, Singapore, Johannesburg, and Taiwan offer services similar to those in the United States for cardiology patients who must undergo angioplasty and bypass surgeries. Individuals with nervous system and neurology disorders may consider hospitals in the Czech Republic, Israel, Guatemala, and Canada. People with orthopedic health issues, such as hip replacements, knee replacements, or bone-related diseases, may consider treatment in Japan, China, or Italy but also are watching Brazil and India as up-and-comers in orthopedic treatments.

The reasons range from access to stem cell treatment to lower costs, blended with an atmosphere that eagerly seeks cash-paying patients. Bring along family members to help you recover in a setting that would typically be just for vacationers.

In response to foreign medical services, American hospitals also have positioned themselves as destinations for out-of-country patients who seek similar services. Today, many more foreign patients are coming to U.S. hospitals because they can get treatment faster than they may in their own country.

But is medical tourism safe? Not so fast, say some medical societies who warn patients of potential complications. Consumers should investigate the hospital's record for post-procedure infections and use of unregulated and potentially unsafe presciption dosages. Know the costs before you commit, including your hotel expenses if you determine that treatment will be done during peak season or if you need to extend your stay due to complications. Also consider patient and family safety should medical tourism be on your mind and budget.

The Medical Travel Commission established patient certification criteria designed to recognize health care organizations that provide extraordinary "best in class service to patients traveling across international borders for care." The inspection process includes seventy-two proprietary criteria, ranging from in-person and phone interviews, documentation review, and evaluation of policies and programs before they receive the MTC seal of approval.

If you are considering treatment in another country, go through a medical travel agency that will help navigate hotel rooms that also accommodate patient-centered care with nurses who will come to your room and care for the patient during your stay. A medical travel agency also will assist in scheduling appointments for consultations and surgical procedures.

First timers should begin by using a U.S.-based medical travel agency such as MedRetreat, read the *Medical Tourism Magazine*, or look for agencies that are members in good standing with the Medical Tourism Association.

Are You a Candidate for Clinical Trials?

Your physician may recommend you for a clinical trial, or you may seek one on your own. The National Institutes of Health offers good guidance on clinical research and questions you should ask before participating.

The best first step to determine whether there is a clinical trial for your disease category is to talk to your doctor. New trials are constantly being created.

The Center for Information and Study on Clinical Research Participation (CIS-CRP) offers an online clinical trials search engine as well as a toll-free number you can call to help find a clinical trial. Or call 1-877 MED HERO if you want to talk to a live person.

Cool Tools

- **Finding a Clinical Trial** is a list of at least eight sources that you can search to learn if there is a trial for your disease.

- **Clinical Trials Mobile App** is supported by the National Library of Medicine and maintains a local study that matches specified categories and key words.

- **Nursing Home Compare** shows you how to compare one nursing home with another. For example, you may want to know how many beds are in one nursing home over another. This may help inform you on how much socialization your loved one may receive. You also want to know credentialing details of the nurses, who is the chief medical officer, how many patients have experienced pressure sores (formerly called bedsores), or how many patients contracted urinary tract infections or experience incontinence. This site also provides details on what's included in a nursing home inspection and how to report a problem to authorities who will act on your complaint if your loved one's care has been compromised. Remember that if treatment requires long-term rehabilitation, your second opinion should include background research on skilled nursing facilities and rehabilitation centers.

- Hospital Compare answers the question, "Is this a safe hospital for me or my loved one?" Data measure hospitals' effectiveness for treating stroke, blood clots, pregnancy and delivery, hospital-acquired infection rates, and readmission rates. The authors reference this website frequently, especially if a friend or family is concerned about the care they are likely to experience. Always check the hospital's HA-MRSA score before entering a hospital. HA-MRSA stands for "hospital-acquired methicillin-resistant staphylococcus aureus" infection, a potentially deadly bacterium that is resistant to most antibiotics. MRSA is usually preventable with cleaners, disinfectants, sanitizers, and the effective use of latex gloves.

- Hospital spending comparisons help inform patients and families what treatments cost at various facilities. This is one of our favorite websites for nearly all treatments because it offers spending comparisons for procedures nationwide and provides the real cost for Medicare reimbursement. If you are a self-paying patient, this information is invaluable to help you negotiate payment.

- Medical Tourism provides guidance to learn more about what countries and regions specialize in surgical procedures or treatment plans.

- Until 2014, infertility clinics were the only clinical specialties required to report their success rate. In 2015, physicians will begin reporting clinical data to the Centers for Medicare and Medicaid Services. Until then, consumers typically reference the following websites for consumer experiences with their health care providers.

  - Lifescript.com, for women looking for a healthier lifestyle, provides guidance on exercise myths and tips; foods designed for women; disease-specific maintenance tips; exercise plans for strength building, toning, and flexibility, depending on your fitness level; celebrity diets; and cosmetic and aging tips. The site is advertising driven, and advertisers pay for each click-through.

- Healthgrades.com provides guidance on how to find a physician or hospital based on findings reported back by patients. Physicians and hospitals have a love–hate relationship with Healthgrades because they prefer to be measured by clinical outcomes rather than the patient experience. But they also realize that patients are the source of new business. As a result, providers and their public relations agencies pay attention to Healthgrades ratings. Search for a physician by condition (e.g., breast cancer, endometriosis, fibromyalgia, or multiple sclerosis), by procedure (e.g., anterior cruciate ligament (ACL) surgery, bariatric surgery, or dermabrasion), or by specialty (cardiology, endocrinology, or nephrology). Let's say you are searching for a provider who treats fibromyalgia. If you selected this from the list of conditions, you will find a list of doctors, with the highest star ratings listed first, who are closest to your location. Read the responses. We prefer responses from fifteen or more users for a more accurate assessment. Be sure to click on the doctor's name to learn about his or her board certifications. For example, if you are seeking help for fibromyalgia, you want a physician certified in rheumatology and internal medicine. Healthgrades also coordinates background information from the past five years, for example, from medical board actions, sanctions, and malpractice claims (if attorneys haven't first removed them from public viewing).

- Vitals.com, similar to Healthgrades, is an online search engine that can help you find a physician by specialty, location, condition, insurance, and urgent care centers. Vitals also tracks the medical practice's performance so that you can anticipate wait time and see if staff are courteous and lets you know if this doctor is accepting new patients. As with Healthgrades, Vitals allows you to also view awards, such as the Patients' Choice Award and Compassionate Doctor Recognition, as well as the medical associations the physician reports he or she is a member of. Vitals also offers a look at the insurance plans accepted by the practice.

- Leapfrog Hospital Survey Results: The Leapfrog Group is a voluntary program that helps employers make informed decisions about health care safety, quality, and customer value. The Leapfrog Hospital Safety Score assigns A, B, C, D, and F grades to more than 2,500 U.S. hospitals based on their ability to prevent errors, accidents, injuries, and infections.

- One of the newer websites on the block is Ucomparehealthcare.com. At this site, you can compare physicians whose profile has been searched the most ("Today's Top Trending Doctors" and "This Week's Top Trending Doctors"). Trending doctors can be for positive and not-so-positive reasons. Select one physician from a list by state, view that physician's profile, and then select another physician for comparison. This tool is best used if you know the names of the physicians you want to compare. Before setting an appointment, we also recommend that you visit their website.

- WebMD.com is one of the most popular search sites for consumer education. Search for physicians at Doctor.webmd.com. The same data offered at Healthgrades and Vitals are also offered at WebMD (largely because they all tap into the same data research engine). The advantage of using this site is that you can quickly conduct additional patient-specific research at the same website and then look for a physician who can treat a condition.

- Looking for a discount on a new prescription? Try a search at helprx.info/discounts. Discounts at this site range from a low of 82 percent off to a high of 91 percent. These represent drugs where the manufacturer offers discounts through the National Prescription Savings Network. Most likely, your pharmacy will ask for your Rx Savings Card, which you can also obtain at the same site. The catch here is that to claim your discount, your insurance prescription benefits plan will, in real time, cross-check benefits to ensure that you are eligible for the discounted price. If you are uninsured or your insurance does not cover prescription drugs, mention this site to your physician to see if you can get an alternative drug that is covered under this national network.

Key Takeaways

In this chapter, you learned the following:

- The value of a second opinion.
- Sometimes a second opinion is requested by the insurance company and sometimes by a physician.
- You also have the right to request another opinion, as it may be exactly what you need to feel comfortable in the treatment to come.

In chapter 3, we focus on how to combine medical, insurance, and family history details into your personal health record and keep it secure. The next time a physician hands you a pile of paperwork to complete, you can hand them your personal health record. The format is the same, but some doctors are just learning how to support patients with these records.

03 Build Your Patient and Family Records

Of all the tools provided in this book, the personal health record (PHR) is your most important tool. We devoted this entire chapter to helping you compile your PHR in a standardized format used by doctors, hospitals, nursing homes, and urgent care facilities in the United States. PHRs save lives, especially in the emergency room, where information is critical within a very short amount of time.

Your PHR is similar to a debit card. In the financial world, you can use your debit card at online and retail stores and to obtain cash at banks where you may or may not have an account. In the health care world, your PHR alerts physicians to your current medications, diseases, members of your care team, and insurance plan. As with your debit card, you are responsible for its security, so we address security measures as well.

In this chapter, we provide guidance on the following:

- What a PHR is.
- How PHRs are time-savers and lifesavers.
- What information should be included in the PHR.
- What PHR is right for you.
- How to secure your PHRs on a mobile app.

I've waited fifteen years to write this book and especially this chapter. When I personally saw the intense need for PHRs, the infrastructure was not there. Provider networks, wires, connections, standards—not even a desire for PHRs was on the minds of providers, but they were on the minds of caregivers. When my brother was fighting pancreatic cancer and his body was traumatized by complications from his chemotherapy mix and painkillers, the emergency room physicians administered larger doses of pain medications, inadvertently adding to his delirium because they didn't have access to his medical history. When my sister was battling brain cancer, my brother- in-law carried his paper notebook between providers, schlepping clinical findings between providers so that the physician-at-the-moment-of-care could access results of her blood tests or daily updates to her medications. When my dad was admitted to a nursing home, he also stopped speaking to the family, including my legally blind mother. She regularly mailed paperwork to me to complete, scan, and send back to the practice, as I was his legal durable power of attorney. When my mom battled T-cell leukemia near the end of her life, a few standards and interfaces were in place, enabling me to intercept her lab results and call her doctor 1,500 miles away to let him know she was crashing and needed a blood transfusion. All too often, a caregiver is the patient's primary advocate.

I built electronic versions of my brother's, my sister's, my father's, and my mother's PHRs, but at no time could any physician access them electronically. Not that the physician didn't want to. The technology infrastructure wasn't there. Even when I printed out hard copies for Mom and Dad, the paper format wasn't compatible with the order the front desk was accustomed to receiving, and I still got that time-consuming clipboard of papers to complete, even though I had everything they needed to provide care and get paid for, just not in "their order."

For the last decade, Peter and I have worked with notable organizations to build and support secure electronic exchange of confidential health information in a consistent format. We became part of a network of industry leaders in small (sometimes loud) ways, helping the federal government, public and private payers (insurance companies), software developers, physician medical groups, legislators, and industry associations toil through competitive and proprietary communication exchanges so that you could get to this chapter in *The Caregiver's Toolbox* and build your own PHR. Our hope is that your PHR will be a time-saver and a lifesaver for you and your loved ones.

(Carolyn Hartley)

What's with Your Doctor's Sign-In Paperwork?

You know the drill. Make an appointment to see the doctor. Fill out paperwork. Wait until the front office builds a record from your information before you are called back into the clinic. See the nurse. Wait. Few doctors now ask, "Why are you here?," as that is a signal that the nurse and doctor are not communicating. The question was intended to build a rapport with you, but after completing six pages of information, you would think someone could have informed your doctor of why you are here.

Those were the old days. Today's doctor provides new patient forms on the practice's website or mails them out to you prior to your visit. You complete the registration form with details about your reason for the visit and medical history and provide surgical and medication background information. You may be asked to send your documents to the practice prior to the visit, but first call to be sure the e-mail exchange is secure. As the caregiver, you provide this same information to each hospital, each lab, and each imaging center. Content in hand, the doctor now says, "Tell me more about your <name of ailment>."

The problem is that each time you complete the paperwork, the content you provide varies, depending on several factors:

- How frustrated you are with the information-gathering process

- Whether you like the doctor and staff

- Whether you can remember how the prescription is really spelled and how many milligrams of a prescription your loved one takes

- Having problems getting it together today

These are all very good reasons, but they create holes in your medical history and put you or your loved one's safety at risk. Save time, save trees, and be consistent with your information by creating a single source document, your PHR, and storing it in a secure place.

What Is a PHR?

A PHR is a technology platform that consumers use to get engaged in their own health care. PHRs are mobile apps that help you build and track data without the help of your physician. Later in this chapter, we discuss patient portals that are offered by your physician, but in this section, we focus on you and your PHR.

The PHR is an electronic record that is built and owned by you, the consumer/patient. The electronic health record (EHR) is owned and managed by the medical practitioner at a hospital, practice, or urgent care facility. Clinical information from the EHR can be securely downloaded into your PHR when both you and the physician agree on security measures that protect both the physician's electronic charts and your PHR. We will take a look at those security issues at the end of this chapter.

PHRs fall into two categories: (1) those protected by the organization that gave it to you, such as your employer or health plan, and (2) those you must protect yourself, usually free or available for a small annual fee.

Regarding the first category, your employer may offer a PHR as part of its benefits package. For example, your employer may be self-insured and offer a PHR so that you can track your health history and those for whom you pay a monthly health care premium. A health insurance company, such as Blue Cross Blue Shield, AETNA, Cigna, Humana, or TriCare, may also provide you with a PHR. In most cases, these PHRs are available to you through a Web portal that they host. In order to access your PHR, you would be required to have a unique user ID and password to verify that you are the correct person.

In this category, your employer or health plan must protect your personal health information using a combination of firewalls and powerful antivirus software to protect your information from malicious attack. Once you download health information from the safety of this portal into an application on your smartphone or mobile device or even print it on paper, it is no longer the responsibility of your employer or health plan to protect the information on your device. Now it is your responsibility to protect your medical information. The employer or health plan will continue to secure any protected health information on its Web portal but is no longer required to protect information that you store on your devices.

In the second category, you are the owner of the PHR. You either downloaded it for free or purchased a PHR app for your smartphone, mobile device, or computer that allows you to track family health information, appointments, medication refill reminders, access to legal documents, access to medical information in emergencies, and much more. Cool Tools at the end of this chapter provide in-depth reviews of widely used and secure PHRs.

How Should I Build My PHR?

You may need one to three hours to compile your medical history into a PHR. Consider this experience to be significant patient safety activity and a cost saver. The variable is that sometimes physicians and hospitals can be a little testy about giving you your own information, but there are laws on your side. We tackle these in chapter 8. The good news is that as of 2015, all health care providers who are using certified electronic medical record software must follow one standard format. If you are a techie, this standard is the Consolidated Clinical Document Architecture (C-CDA). In table 3.1, we provide that format in plain language along with tips on how to find what you need.

Gather the details first, and then we will present Cool Tools for storing your content.

Table 3.1. Building Your PHR: What You Need and Where to Find It

Directions: Check the completed box when you have gathered information for each line item.

What You Need	What This Means and Where to Find It	Completed?
Patient name	This is your legal name. Women, you can put your maiden name in parentheses unless your legal name provided on your Social Security registration includes your maiden name.	❑
Insurance information	Insurance information is not part of the C-CDA, but it is the first question all health care organizations ask before delivering care. Important insurance information includes the following: *Your name*	❑
	Name of subscriber: This is the person in your family who pays for the coverage. If insurance is offered by your employer and you have authorized a monthly deduction to cover health care costs, you are the subscriber. If you are covered under your spouse's plan, your spouse is the subscriber. Subscriber may also be called "Member."	
	Subscriber ID: This is the number on your insurance card typically found immediately below the subscriber's name.	
	Effective date: This is the date your insurance became effective.	
	Group number: This number refers to the employer's group policy.	
Emergency contacts	Provide the name and phone number of the person you want the provider to call if there is an emergency. While you are gathering this information, also add your emergency contacts into your smartphone's ICE (In Case of Emergency) group.	❑
Sex	Male, female	❑
Date of birth	Most people know this.	❑

(continued)

Table 3.1. *(continued)*

What You Need	What This Means and Where to Find It	Completed?
Race	Race is Caucasian, African American, Hispanic, Asian, American Indian, and so on. Race refers to a person's physical appearance, for example, skin color, eye color, hair color, and bone/jaw structure. *Why does my doctor need this?* The Agency for Healthcare Research and Quality (AHRQ) finds that some races receive worse care than others and that some diseases are more likely to occur among specific races. In 2050, AHRQ estimates racial groups other than Caucasian will account for half of the U.S. population. Public health agencies hope to eliminate health disparities and also anticipate delivery of care for these populations. By analyzing these data, AHRQ can provide more consistent medical treatment regardless of your race.	❏
Ethnicity	Ethnicity refers to cultural factors, such as nationality, ancestry, language, and beliefs or a shared group history. You may be Irish, Welsh, German, French, Chinese, Korean, Scandinavian, Asian, Middle Eastern, Hispanic, and so on. *Why does my doctor need this?* Similar to AHRQ's research, the Institute of Medicine (IOM) has concluded in its studies that "racial and ethnic disparities in health care exist with greater morbidity and mortality from chronic diseases" among people of some ethnicities. This means that because of your ethnicity, you may not be receiving the care you deserve. By tracking how health care is delivered, IOM and public health agencies hope to eliminate health care disparities.	❏
Preferred language	Most frequently reported are English, Spanish, French, and Chinese. Your doctor may be bilingual and choose to communicate with you in your language.	❏
Care team members	Your care team members include the following: 1. Your doctor's name, practice's address, and phone number. a. Begin with your primary care or internal medicine provider's name.	❏

What You Need	What This Means and Where to Find It	Completed?
	b. Add a specialist or specialists after your primary care physician.	
	c. Some women view their gynecologist as their primary physician. That's fine.	
	2. The doctor's nurse's name, practice's address, and phone number. Most caregivers know the nurse's name, names of children, where they live, where they play soccer, and where they were last Saturday night. Keep it simple with just the nurse's name, phone number, and address.	
	3. If you are the patient's appointed caregiver, include your name as a member of the care team. For example, as the caregiver, you may be the spouse, son, or daughter, and your loved one has signed the practice's authorization that it is okay to communicate details about care and treatment with you. If you are not the spouse, you will need legal documentation to support your role as a member of the care team. A durable power of attorney document is required in most states.	
	4. If you are the parent or legal guardian of a minor (0–18 years), you should be included in the care team. In the event of a divorce or legal separation, the person holding primary custody is listed as a member of the care team. Keep track of court documents in the event you must verify that you are the custodial parent. The PHRs we recommend provide the capability to upload and store online documents and files.	
Allergies	1. Begin with allergic reactions to medications.	❏
	a. Identify your reaction (hives, rash, swollen eyes, throat swelling, heart palpitations, seizures, anaphylaxis, etc.).	
	b. On a scale of 1 to 10, identify the severity of the reaction.	
	2. List environmental allergies, such as allergy to pollen, pet dander, wheat, corn, and so on.	
	a. Identify your reaction (hives, rash, swollen eyes, throat swelling, coughing attacks, heart palpitations, etc.)	
	b. On a scale of 1 to 10, identify the severity of the reaction.	

(continued)

Table 3.1. *(continued)*

What You Need	What This Means and Where to Find It	Completed?

Medications	Open your medicine cabinet, your vitamin shelf, and your handbag to build this list.
	
	1. Begin with your current prescription medications.
	   a. Add the name of the medication, the dosage, and the route by which you take the medication (by mouth, suppository, injection, topical, etc.).
	   b. Add medications you used to take in the past three years, especially if they caused a reaction or a long-lasting side effect.
	2. Add the over-the-counter drugs you take on a regular basis.
	   a. This includes daily low-dose aspirin, pain management drugs, sleeping aids, allergy medications, weight loss herbal teas, injections or pills, acne pills or lotions, pills to stop smoking, laxatives, and so on.
	3. Add your vitamins and herbal supplements.
	   a. This includes daily multivitamins, fish oil, herbal supplements for depression, heart health, energy, metabolism, and so on. *Why does your doctor need to know?* Vitamins may cause an interaction with medications you are taking. Consult MedlinePlus if you are concerned about any interactions between herbal supplements and your prescribed medications.
	4. Recreational drugs. Your doctor is unlikely to turn your loved one in to the police, but the doctor does need to know if the patient is taking drugs to help manage the pain, depression, or anxiety. Marijuana, ecstasy, methadone, and PCP, for example, alter the effectiveness of prescription medication. Sometimes the interaction can be deadly.
		❏

Care plan	Your care plan is also the treatment plan that your doctor is recommending and that you agreed to follow or are at least attempting to follow. Your care plan is likely to include one or a combination of several diagnostic tools and treatments.	❏

What You Need	What This Means and Where to Find It	Completed?
	Diagnostic Tools	
	• Biopsy	
	• Regular blood or urine tests	
	• Images, such as sonograms, bone density (dexascans), mammograms, CT scans, and PET scans	
	• X-rays, such as a chest X-ray	
	• Care Plan (Treatment)	
	• Prescription medication	
	• Physical therapy	
	• Referral to a specialist	
	• One or more surgical procedures	
	• Diet, nutrition plan, and exercise	
	• Educational material	
	• Psychological support	
	• Mobility equipment	
	Your care plan may include products to help keep your loved one mobile. For example, you may need a seeing-eye dog, a wheelchair or walker, or hearing-assisted or speech-assisted tools. Your doctor may recommend that you find mobility support locally. Several organizations have compiled detailed links to other resources. Three sites to consider include these:	
	• Able Data for helping adults	
	• Adventures in Movement for the Handicapped (AIM) for helping children	
	• Rosalynn Carter Institute for Caregiving for helping children and adults	

(continued)

Table 3.1. *(continued)*

What You Need	What This Means and Where to Find It	Completed?
	If your physician uses certified EHR technology (ONC-certified software embedded inside the computer), the good news is that you should receive a "clinical summary" or "patient visit summary" at the end of each visit. This summary includes all of the items above. Your patient summary also may be provided for you in the practice's patient portal. More on patient portals in this chapter.	
	As time permits, keep a journal of how your loved one's body is responding to the care plan.	
Problem list	The problem list is your diagnosis.	☐
	1. Begin with your most current diagnosis.	
	Most doctors are direct and provide you with details about the problems your loved one's body is managing. If you feel your doctor isn't giving you enough details, you can look at the bill the office handed to you and that said, "Take this to checkout as you leave." In order to get paid, your doctor must identify a diagnosis and a treatment plan. Your diagnosis is either circled or written in the lower right side of the bill. Write down that number, and when you get home, look up the number online. Begin your search with "ICD," followed by the number. (ICD stands for International Classification of Diseases.) We get into more detail on this in chapter 7.	
	Most caregivers find their loved ones have multiple problems, such as diabetes, high blood pressure, and Alzheimer's. Some problems are more obvious some days than others. The diagnoses for this field are the ones that your doctor has identified, not the ones you think are a problem.	
	2. What if you find other problems?	

What You Need	What This Means and Where to Find It	Completed?
	Say you find that your loved one begins coughing at night, but you cannot tell if it's heartburn, nocturnal asthma, or gastroesophageal reflux disorder. Keep track of these additional symptoms so that you can bring them to the doctor's attention in your next visit unless you feel the symptoms require urgent attention. In that case, call 911 for emergency help.	
Laboratory tests and results	In this section, store the results of your lab tests, sonograms, X-rays, biopsies, or scans. You probably won't have space to store the digital image, as these take up considerable space. However, the lab or imaging center sent a copy of the results to your physician, and you are entitled as either a caregiver or a patient to receive a copy of that report. Most physicians now print a copy of these reports for you without your having to ask for them. Some doctors still need a little training, so ask away!	❏
Procedures (surgical history)	Like most Americans, you've been to multiple hospitals for surgical procedures. It's unlikely that the hospitals have shared details of those surgeries with other hospitals unless you or your doctor specifically directed them to do so. This means that you are the resource for health information exchange. In this section, list the most current procedures first. If you recall the month and year, you are doing better than most readers. Do not fret over surgeries done more than ten years ago unless they are part of your current problem. For example, if you have been cancer free for ten years and a new spot appears on another part of your body, your oncologist will want to know about your previous surgeries.	❏
Smoking status	Do you smoke? How many packs a day? Are you a former smoker? How long did you smoke before quitting? If you are a nonsmoker, simply say, "Nonsmoker."	❏

(continued)

Table 3.1. *(continued)*

What You Need	What This Means and Where to Find It	Completed?
Vital signs	Enter numbers that are most current for the following:	❑
	Height.	
	Weight.	
	Temperature when not sick.	
	Blood pressure (systolic and diastolic). This changes during the day, but you should know your averages.	
	Glucose level—especially important for individuals with diabetes.	
	Cholesterol—both LDL (bad) and HDL (good).	
Family medical history	Most doctors are interested in knowing diseases in your immediate family. They also want to know if your loved one's parents are still living and, if deceased, the age when they passed.	❑
	Mother	
	Father	
	Brother	
	Sister	
	Grandmother	
	Grandfather	
Advance directives	Do your loved ones have an advance directive? This is a legal document that tells health care professionals and family members about treatment preferences for termination of life support and organ donation in the event the individual is not able to make such a decision.	❑

PHRs: Selection "Must-Haves"

When considering a PHR for you or your caregiver, consider the PHR comparison tool in table 3.2 for your must-haves. To complete the comparison tool, print this chart and take notes as you review one or more of the PHRs that follow. Notice that some of the PHRs are disease specific. Use the "Must-Haves" sections to determine if the PHR meets your requirements.

Table 3.2. PHR Comparison Tool

Must-Haves	PHR #1 _____	PHR #2 _____	PHR #3 _____
Accessible through smartphone, Dropbox, and online			
Organizes family health information			
Scans documents into the PHR using your camera			
Builds trend lines to track conditions			
Sets unlimited medication reminders			
Sets appointment reminders that interface with your own schedule			
Adds files from other apps and from your computer			
Exports documents and imports them into your PHR			
Stores medications and allergies information			
E-mails summaries or graphs to your doctor			
Tracks insurance information and reimbursements			
Provides a symptoms checker			
Available in multiple languages			

PHRs for Your Review and Selection

Many PHRs that are free are also supported by advertisers seeking your business. In building your PHR, consider the services that the company may offer against getting a free PHR.

Microsoft HealthVault

Microsoft HealthVault is the largest of all the PHR companies and also connects with more than 230 mobile devices. This means that mobile devices owned by companies like Bayer, Carematix, Microlife, Fitbit, Nipro, Omron, Polar, Sinovo, and many others have developed a link that connects and stores information into your HealthVault PHR. For example, a patient managing diabetes can use a glucose-monitoring device that links its device with HealthVault. Similar devices track blood pressure or walking distance. At Healthvault.com, you will find a list of devices that connect with this PHR. As a caregiver, you receive immediate results from the device, but when uploaded into your HealthVault PHR, you can monitor results over time.

Some company PHRs also use HealthVault PHR as the back end of their PHR but rebrand it as their own. LabCorp, the American Cancer Society, LiveHealthier, NextofKin Registry, and nearly 150 other mobile apps link to HealthVault. Many doctors and hospitals also use HealthVault as a link to their patient portals. Be sure to create an emergency profile for your loved one if this is the PHR you choose.

There is no fee to consumers for using HealthVault. This application is often selected by younger, healthier audiences.

Capzule PHR by Webahn

Capzule PHR continually shows up on the top five lists of PHR reviews. In addition to keeping your own medical record, you can also record details about your family members on Capzule PHR. Features include pill reminders and glucose and blood pressure tracking with charts to quickly see trends with immunization and medication records. You can track insurance lists and physician portal messages. Capzule PHR also supports photos of caregivers so that emergency personnel can confirm that they have the correct information for your loved one. It is an attractive PHR with broad consumer appeal. Upload documents from multiple sources into Capzule PHR and electronically share them with family members if you choose.

This app connects with Google Drive, Dropbox, Walgreens, and HealthVault. It costs $2.95 to download online onto your smartphone or $4.95 from your iTunes library. It is compatible with iPhone and iPad.

iTriageHealth

The iTriageHealth app is a powerful PHR designed by emergency room physicians. Originally developed to be a symptoms checker and to redirect patients who didn't need to be in the emergency room to the pharmacy, iTriageHealth now has expanded to be a medical book in the palm of your hand.

When using iTriageHealth, you can check trends to give you a look at the top ten currently reported diseases in the area. Using the symptoms checker available in alphabetical order or by clicking on a male or female avatar, you can get a list of pains and conditions with related images, videos, and resources to connect in your area. Instantly find directions to hospitals, poison control centers, and urgent care facilities. If you are scheduled for a procedure, look it up on iTriageHealth to obtain a broad to detailed description, videos of the procedure, and follow-up care.

The My iTriage component stores your health information, including insurance, medications, and dosages. iTriageHealth is used frequently by parents and families.

iBlueButton

iBlueButton is a federal initiative that began as a PHR for veterans and expanded to Medicare and Medicaid recipients. iBlueButton also conforms to the C-CDA requirements. After several years of being available only to federal employees, the Office of the National Coordinator decided to broaden access to the general public. Using iBlueButton, you can securely access and exchange EHRs, including X-ray images and reports, lab results, and clinical summaries. Your physician may be using iBlueButton Professional, and an iBlueButtonVeterans is available for veterans. Caregivers supporting an aging population find that many providers access iBlueButton with greater frequency than other PHRs.

NoMoreClipboard

NoMoreClipboard is one of the surviving PHR companies that entered the marketplace in the mid-2000s and then broadened its reach into academic medical centers and hospitals. Since it is linked to HealthVault, you can get a free PHR from NoMoreClipboard.

If you are looking for a PHR that provides additional services to you, consider one of the plans that range from $9.95 to $119.95 per year. The advantage of a costlier PHR is that NoMoreClipboard sends registration forms to the physicians you indicate before you arrive in the waiting room. We think this is a bit pricey, but many caregivers prefer the ease of having forms completed before arriving at the practice or hospital.

NavigatingCancer

PHR systems have a difficult time competing with the thoroughness of Navigating Cancer. This PHR is the most advanced tool for individuals and their caregivers managing cancer and blood disorders.

At Navigating Cancer, you can access nearly 200 chemotherapy drug articles and the types of cancers each drug is used to treat. You also will find discussion groups from patients and their caregivers offering advice on how to manage home care, how to build your survivorship plan, and how to connect with other individuals and families in treatment for the same cancers your loved one is managing. An oncologist once said, "No patients are more educated on their disease than patients with cancer." Navigating Cancer seeks to keep families fighting cancer deeply involved in the education and treatment loop. Navigating Cancer is used by a large majority of oncology practices as their patient portal and is free to consumers/patients and caregivers.

Health and Health Kit

Health, by Apple, is a relative newcomer to the health apps scene and may be one of the caregiver's most comprehensive tools. Still early in consolidating health information from multiple resources, the Health Kit app promises to help caregivers store medical information downloaded from multiple physicians into a single file.

CareConnector

Offered by the Johnson & Johnson Caregiver initiative, CareConnector includes a Care Planner to store insurance, health care provider names, emergency contact information, a prescription tracker and medication history, and a message board to communicate with other caregivers.

Secure Your PHR

While PHRs bring together multiple resources to help you as a caregiver, they also present a risk that you might accidentally expose your confidential health information to others. You don't want someone to steal your identity and obtain medical services using your insurance information, nor do you want someone outside your immediate family to participate in your care unless you specifically give them access. Let's talk about best practices:

1. Your smartphone should be accessible only with a user ID and password.
2. The PHR you store on your smartphone or mobile device must be accessed with a user ID and password. Do not allow your smartphone to automatically save this sensitive information. Log in every time.

3. Consider incoming texts, images, or requests to download an application as threats from someone trying to gain access to your information. For example, "Click on this link, and you'll have access to thousands of free ringtones" sounds too good to be true because it is a malicious link from an organization trying to gain access to your personal information.

4. Update your operating system. Updates provide enhanced functionality and new features, and they also include fixes to critical security vulnerabilities. Your smartphone manufacturer will notify you when an update is available.

5. Use security software. Our favorites are Lookout, Avast!, ESET, and Avira, as each of these had a 100 percent virus detection rate in Digital Trend's AV-Test. As news continues to pour in about cybercrime's ties to Eastern Europe, avoid downloading security software manufactured in those countries. If your smartphone contains confidential information and is lost or stolen, our favorite software packages mentioned here will wipe your phone clean and provide you with a location finder. Be sure you have backed up your data before wiping it clean or evaluate the risks if your data are stolen. Mobile security apps range from free to $2.99 per month.

Patient Portals: The Good, the Bad, and the Really Cool

Has your doctor's office or hospital asked you to sign up for their patient portal? Many insurance companies also offer patient portals, and some will send you a bonus check if you update your medical history.

The Good

Patient portals allow health care professionals to perform many customer-friendly services. Using your doctor's patient portal, you can do the following:

- Request a prescription refill.

- Look for an open spot on the calendar and ask for an appointment.

- Access diagnostic test results, such as from a lab test. Doctors rarely post biopsy results unless they first discuss the results with you.

- Find educational material about your loved one's procedure.

- Find organizations that offer support to families managing similar diseases.

- Read and respond to blogs from your physician.

- Find answers to common problems after surgeries and signs to watch that indicate your loved one may have a postsurgical infection.

- Allow you to view whether the practice is behind schedule.

If you choose to communicate with your clinical team through the patient portal, look for terms that indicate how quickly a health care professional will respond to your inquiry. Patient portals are not to be used for emergencies, but they are an excellent resource if you need general guidance or a non–urgent care response.

The Bad

Most caregivers bring their loved ones to multiple appointments with different physicians, rehabilitation or infusion centers, and hospitals. Each organization sponsors its own patient portal. Federal government standards-setting organizations are building blocks that will eventually allow patient portals to "talk" to each other, but putting that in place involves approval and adoption from multiple organizations.

The Really Cool

Patient portals that integrate with physician's EHR systems are now releasing a mobile app that looks, acts, and feels like a PHR. For example, you can download the app to your smartphone, secure it with a user ID and password, and then access information when you need it.

The really cool part is that patient portals are tied directly to your physician's or specialist's EHR. You don't have to do all the work building a PHR because information you provide is downloaded into your PHR. You only have to securely sign up to access medications and medical and surgical history, and you can add information if you forgot to tell the physician. Most portals allow you to request a prescription refill, schedule an appointment, or ask the doctor to call you if it isn't an emergency.

Portals now also allow you to sync data from medical devices, such as your glucose meter, blood pressure devices, or wearables, such as Fitbit or Jawbone.

Your physician's practice selects the patient portal because it securely interfaces with their EHR. If you see multiple physicians within the same health system, any physician can send updates into your patient portal or add information to the patient portal, allowing you to compile an electronic resource. You, however, have final approval on what is accepted into your portal record. Consumers using patient portals cannot yet fully experience the interoperability benefits they have with debit cards. For example, you can swipe your debit card at nearly every bank in America whether it's yours or not. Hospitals, physicians, and imaging centers within the same health network are now more likely to coordinate your health information to your patient portal. American standards-setting organizations are working diligently to ensure that your PHR can be swiped at every hospital, clinic, surgical center, and urgent care and long-term care facility by 2017.

Key Takeaways

In this chapter, you learned the following:

- A PHR is an application that stores your health information so that you can access it readily without searching through paper documents.

- Be sure to secure your PHR with strong passwords or encryption, as it contains sensitive and confidential information.

- Register for a patient portal when you go into the physician's practice so that you can easily access your health information and health information for your loved one. Obtain your own user ID and password to access your loved one's patient portal account.

- Select a PHR that is right for you and your loved one using the guidance in table 3.2.

04 | Begin Building Your Technology Plan

In this chapter, we begin to build a plan for safeguarding your financial information. Building this technology plan includes putting security measures in place so that sensitive information is accessed only by those authorized to access it. This also includes education on prevention and anti-identity theft measures that protect you and your loved ones against security breaches, such as those from Target and Neiman Marcus in 2013. This chapter also helps shape discussions and identifies what remains to be collected.

In this chapter, we provide guidance on the following:

- What a technology plan is and who needs one.
- How to manage password protection.
- How to manage your personal and financial information.

What Is a Technology Plan?

A technology plan is a layered process that preserves, protects, and manages the individual's "digital legacy." A digital legacy is what you call the compilation of the technology you use every day to make your life run more smoothly. It's more than just accessing e-mail and Facebook; it's using e-banking and online bill payment options, managing investments and memberships, and anything that deals with tracking your personal assets. Information is readily available at your fingertips with the use of computers, but it is vitally important that you assist loved ones in keeping up with the challenges that the use of technology brings.

Who Needs a Technology Plan?

Every person who utilizes the computer needs a technology plan. Likewise, every caregiver needs a technology plan for his or her loved one.

One of the most important challenges you face is safely keeping an up-to-date record of every account with its user name and password. This information needs to be readily available and protected in a secure environment in the event your loved one depends on you to be the caregiver not only for personal and health reasons but also for financial and legal reasons.

"Living 'paperless' seems good until the survivors or caregivers have to seek out and recreate all of the online information that was not documented in a useful manner," says the chief operating officer of a multistate health care network who was the caretaker for her husband. Your goal is to preserve, protect, and manage your loved one's digital information. This is not a simple process.

Use table 4.1 to identify accounts that require user names and passwords.

My dad was the computer person in the house who controlled investments and stocks, while my mom handled the checkbook for day-to-day bills. There was a method to their madness in how they divided and conquered. When Dad had a stroke and lost his short-term memory, our family became painfully aware that Mom knew none of the user names and passwords to their accounts. She could not even log on to their computer without this information. This opened our eyes to the fact we that we needed a plan. How could we, as caregivers, assist them in managing and preserving their personal and financial information when only Dad knew the passwords to their accounts? Were there other parts of their digital legacy that neither Mom nor we were aware of? We needed an inventory of their accounts in order to put our arms around the situation.

How did we get started? We began by building an inventory of Mom and Dad's accounts. To find more detailed information, we ordered a credit report to get a list of their financial accounts. We reviewed their e-mails, financial statements, and past regular mail. We searched through filing cabinets. We went through their wallets and purses for credit card or membership information. We even scoured the sticky notes and memos surrounding their computer since we knew that many individuals keep user names and passwords in the general area of their computers.

We learned a few lessons that may help you as you build your list of accounts. We learned that proper identification is needed to access accounts: driver's license, Social Security card, membership number, power of attorney, and so on. We learned that each individual needs photo identification and that individuals who no longer drive should still retain a photo driver's license even if it is expired. We also learned the importance of adding the caregiver's name to each account and the importance of having a beneficiary listed on accounts where applicable.

All this enabled us to get a better understanding of our parent's situation and establish a process to access and store their user names and passwords. Thus, we began to build a contingency plan for future similar situations. How much easier this would have been if my parents had used some of the tools we are making available to you.

(Peter Wong)

Table 4.1. Sample Accounts That Require Usernames and Passwords

Name of Account	What Did (Dad/ Mom) Call It?	Where Would We Find It?
Health care accounts		
Health savings accounts		
Insurance accounts		
Computers		
Mobile devices		
Internet services		
Airline memberships		
Car rental memberships		
Hotel memberships		
AARP/AAA memberships		
Television passwords		
Web passwords		
Internet SSID		
Modem passwords to access the Web		
Identity protection services		
Computer backup		
Kindle library		
Frequent shopping sites (eBay, Amazon, etc.)		
iTunes		
Facebook/Twitter/other social media		

Managing Password Protection

Some precautions should be put in place for password storage. For example, if you are using Google Chrome as your Web browser and allowing Chrome to store your passwords, the saved passwords are very easy to access. To test the security of some employees, one software developer simply typed "chrome://settings/pass words" into the Chrome search bar, and all previously stored passwords instantly appeared. He instituted a new policy that day.

Included in Cool Tools are some of the best password manager tools, according to a *Digital Trends* article, "Avoiding Google Chrome Security Flaw with These Password Manager Apps."

There are three basic options for storing passwords:

1. *Memorize them:* Good, effective, but highly unlikely to be useful if your loved one becomes mentally incapable, even for a short amount of time. Also, it is difficult to memorize numerous passwords.
2. *Write them down:* Good and effective (old school), but what if someone finds your list and gains access to your financial information? In spite of many warnings, many Americans still write down passwords and store them on sticky notes under the computer. Sticky notes are very risky and compromise your privacy. You may wish to put them into a password-protected document, but remember the pass code to access them.
3. *Password storage:* Good, effective, easier to manage, but possibly susceptible to risk. The software uses a master password to manage all your passwords. With the right software installed, you need only one password.

Each individual will have to determine which option or combination of options is best.

Cool Tools for Password Protection

- CardStar app imports multiple loyalty cards and access coupons when it's time to check out.

- LastPass 2.0 is a free application (or $12 for more features) and allows you to import all saved passwords from Google Chrome, Firefox, Internet Explorer, Opera, and Safari. LastPass also allows for two-form authentication, such as the YubiKey.

- RoboForm Everywhere stores information locally rather than in the cloud. RoboForm2Go installs on a USB drive rather than the computer's hard drive, allowing the user to take RoboForm on the go.

- 1Password, available for a one-time cost of $50 ($70 for a family license), has an extremely easy-to-use user interface. Many prefer 1Password over LastPass2.0.

Managing Financial Information

Managing financial information is another key component of the technology plan in the caregiver's toolbox. Using technology tools can simplify the management process and provide another safeguard for your loved one. In our experience, the caregiver is faced with two likely scenarios: (1) the loved one wants your involvement, or (2) the loved one does not want your involvement. If you are in the latter situation, there may be a reason why your loved one does not want you in the thick of things. For example, another member of the family is the appointed executor trustee of the estate. Or the financial accounts are stored in a safe-deposit box, and your loved one has listed a trusted friend or other family member as having access to this box. One person must be listed on the bank document and have a key to gain access to the safe-deposit box. A caregiver does not have the right to access the parent's safe-deposit box just because he or she has the power of attorney (defined later in this chapter). *Obtain access to the financial accounts.*

So what do you do if your loved one does not want your involvement in his or her financial situation? It begins with an open discussion that displays love and concern for his or her well-being. It may take having this discussion many times before your loved one recognizes a need for help. It's not easy. Our families have struggled with this dilemma, too. After experiencing deteriorating health and seeing friends go through similar circumstances with their family members, our parents eventually recognized that our help was important and necessary, and we were able to start working together on their financial plan.

Whichever situation you are in, we have found several issues the caregiver must address in order to manage the loved one's financial information:

1. *Locate the financial accounts.*

   The first step is to order a free credit report from each of the three credit score companies—Transunion, Experian, and Equifax—and compare them for consistency. This should be done at least once a year. Schedule time to be with your loved one to explain you are ordering these credit reports to ensure that no unauthorized person has accessed the accounts and also to get a list of all accounts that may be inactive but still listed as an open account. This collaborative discussion will establish and build trust. Not all parents want their children or caregivers "poking" through their personal accounts, so you may need to approach this process several times, continuing to build a trustful relationship to avoid fear from your loved one that you are trying to control or manipulate financial matters. The goal here is not to give financial advice but to simplify financial manageability.

Consider consolidating or closing credit cards for better manageability, as it is not surprising to find ten or more credit cards listed on your loved one's credit report.

According to the National Crime Prevention Council, you should cancel all credit cards or debit cards that have not been used in the past six months. Open credit is a prime target for identity thieves snooping into your credit report.

Also, if possible, consider consolidating financial institutions so there are fewer accounts for the caregiver to track. This will also limit unwanted mail, e-mails, solicitations, and possible fraud or scam exploitations. You are now on your way to building your loved one's accounts inventory.

2. *Obtain access to the financial accounts.*

It is necessary to have the power of attorney in order to manage another's financial accounts. This is a legal document usually drawn up by your loved one's estate attorney when the will was created and signed. The power of attorney authorizes you to handle all banking transactions for your loved one, including depositing and withdrawing money from accounts.

The power of attorney is typically used when your loved one does not have the mental or physical capacity to handle a bank account and works best when there is a high level of trust and understanding between the caregiver and loved one. We will further discuss the power of attorney in chapter 9.

Once you obtain access to the financial accounts, you may find areas that require fine-tuning in order to protect the assets. For example, a common concern the caregiver and loved one share is banking account theft. Having a debit card linked to one's checking account can pose a high risk if the card is stolen or lost. Debit cards may not carry the same level of personal protection as a credit card.

My mom used a debit card and carried a balance of $30,000 in her checking account. She was unaware of her liability in the event her card was lost or stolen. We were very concerned when we realized she kept such a large amount in

Understanding liability in the event of a lost or stolen debit/credit card is important. The Federal Trade Commission is an agency of the federal government established with the principal mission of consumer protection. The commission's mandate is to protect consumers against unfair, deceptive, or fraudulent practices in the marketplace. It provides consumer education information on lost or stolen credit, ATM, or debit cards.

There are many good informational links regarding the use of debit and credit cards. Clark Howard, a noted author and nationally syndicated radio host on consumer protection, offers a review of the places he will never use a debit card. These include the following:

■ Independent ATMs

■ Pay-at-the-pump gas stations

■ Online purchases

■ Restaurants

3. *Ensure that the financial accounts have proper beneficiary and secondary account holders.*

The third step for safeguarding financial accounts is to ensure that the caregiver is listed on the accounts and that the proper beneficiary is also listed on each asset and account. It sounds simple, but it is amazing how many times this step is overlooked. The consequences are frustrating and can be mired in complications.

My father recently passed away. As my brother was going through my mom's paperwork, he discovered a bank account in my father's name that was unknown to her. When he and my mom went to the bank to close the account, they found that Dad had not listed a beneficiary on the account. What could've been a simple banking transaction turned into a complicated matter. We found out that if an account does not list a beneficiary, also known as a payable-on-death provision, the family has to review their legal options, which may include state laws, marital status, and will validation. Because there was no beneficiary listed on this account, Mom had to show proof of marriage to the bank. Normally, at that time the account would be distributed to the estate according to Dad's will. But in our situation, this account was not discovered until six months after Dad's estate had been settled. It is now going through the probate court system for settlement, a much longer process. Thank goodness Mom did not need the money from this account in her near future.

(Peter Wong)

After you have listed a beneficiary on all your accounts, be sure to keep a copy of the documentation for future reference.

4. *Use technology to manage the financial process.*

This is where the Cool Tools help manage the financial process. The tools can assist in organizing and categorizing your loved one's spending. The tools can also pull all the financial information into one place so that you can get an entire picture and stay on top of your loved one's finances (checking, savings, retirement, and investments).

Our family is using some of these tools to help our mom manage her finances. As part of the caregiving team, the tools have given us a greater ability to help Mom organize, track, and pay bills.

(Peter Wong)

After you have identified your loved one's accounts, you can start compiling the information in a table similar to table 4.2.

Table 4.2. Detailed Account Information List

Financial Institution	_____	
Type of Account	Checking account	Account number _____
	Savings account	Account number _____
	Investment account	Account number _____
Brokerage account	Type_____	Account number _____
Power of attorney on file	Yes or no	Date modified _____

Financial Institution	
Address _____	Phone number _____
Name of financial planner _____	
User name _____	
Password _____	
Password hint _____	
Beneficiary _____	

Credit Card Information	Please keep in secure place
Credit card number _____	Expiration date _____
Payment type	Mail in or electronic
Pass code for call in	
Pass code for electronic	
User name _____	
Password _____	
Password hint _____	
Beneficiary _____	

Credit card number _____	Expiration date _____
Payment type	Mail in or electronic
Pass code for call in	
Pass code for electronic	
User name _____	
Password _____	
Password hint _____	
Beneficiary _____	

Other Membership Cards (frequent flyer, AARP, membership programs)	
Member number _____	Expiration date _____
Payment type	Mail in or electronic
Pass code for call in	
Pass code for electronic	
User name _____	

(continued)

Table 4.3. (*continued*)

Other Membership Cards (frequent flyer, AARP, membership programs)	
Password	_____
Password hint	_____
Beneficiary	_____

Home Data Collection	Please keep in secure place

Utility Company	_____
Address	_____
Phone number	_____
Billing cycle date	_____
Payment type	Mail in or electronic

Mortgage Company	
Address	_____
Phone number	_____
Billing cycle date	_____
Payment type	Mail in or electronic
Password for electronic	
User name	_____
Password	_____
Password hint	_____
Beneficiary	_____

Legal Information	Please keep documents in a secure place

Attorney name	_____
Address	_____
Phone number	_____
E-mail address	_____
Specialty area	_____
	(real estate, will, trust, advance directives, power of attorney)

Cool Tools for Managing Financial Information

- Mint.com, a free app available on iPhone or Android, is a finance management program that allows the caregiver to monitor the loved one's financial situation at any time. Mint.com allows for a wide range of assets, such as bank accounts, investment accounts, loans, and real estate. It is a *Money* magazine Top Pick, a Kiplinger Award winner, a Webby Award winner, and a CNN Money Award winner.

- Yodlee MoneyManagement, a free app available on iPhone or Android, is a personal financial management program that helps the caregiver categorize the loved one's spending by tracking accounts. It can be used to pay bills and transfer funds between online bank accounts, credit cards, investment accounts, loans, mortgages, and insurance.

- Hellowallet, also available on iPhone or Android, is a personal financial management app that charges a monthly fee. The online financial guidance service helps you budget and set personal financial goals in addition to tracking and monitoring your transactions.

- Checkme, a free app available on iPhone and Android, is a financial management app used for paying bills, monitoring accounts, and scheduling payments. It is one of *Redbook* magazine's "9 Best Money Apps for 2014," CNBC's "Best Financial Apps 2014," and *PC Magazine*'s "Best Android Apps 2013."

Managing Personal Information

"Your personal information is a valuable commodity. It's not only the key to your financial identity, but also to your online identity," says the Federal Trade Commission. The caregiver needs to stay informed regarding events that may impact the loved one's personal information, such as the recent Heartbleed virus and the 2013 Target data breach. There are many sources of information, but we recommend three:

1. *Federal Bureau of Investigation (FBI):* A federal government agency working to prevent criminal activities to the public.
   FBI Scams/Computer Safety: This is a list of practical guidelines from the FBI regarding how to protect your PC from scams and outside threats to your personal information.

2. *Federal Trade Commission (FTC):* The nation's consumer protection agency that works to prevent fraudulent, deceptive, and unfair business practices

to the marketplace. The FTC provides key tips regarding how to keep the consumer's information secure, along with ways to protect personal information from hackers, online thieves, and other outside threats.

FTC Identity Theft: This website provides immediate guidance on what to do if you believe you or your loved one is a victim of identity theft.

FTC Computer Security: This website provides access to a free and low-cost computer protection products and services. Guard against using free products, as those are the ones the scammers use first to hack into your system.

3. *National Crime Prevention Council (NCPC):* A private nonprofit organization whose mission is to provide consumer information on crime prevention (*NCPC Consumer Guide on Identity Theft*). This is an educational link that

Table 4.3.   Key Numbers to Call If You Have Been a Victim of Identity Theft

Organization	Your Local Number
Contact the U.S. Postal Inspection Service if you suspect that someone has used your mailing address to commit a crime. Call (888) 877-7644 for the number of your local office.	
Contact the Internal Revenue Service if you think your identification has been used in violation of tax laws. Call (800) 829-0433.	
Contact the Social Security Administration if your Social Security number has been stolen. The Fraud Hotline is (800) 269-0271.	
Contact the Federal Trade Commission, which keeps a database that law enforcement agencies use to find identity thieves. Call the toll-free hotline at (877) IDTHEFT.	
If you believe someone has fraudulently opened a checking account in your name, contact Chex Systems at (800) 428-9623. Chexhelp is the consumer reporting service used by many banks; however, if your bank doesn't use Chex Systems, you can ask for the name and number of the consumer reporting service it uses.	
If someone is illegally using your bank account, do the following: 1. Close the account immediately. 2. Have your bank notify its check verification service to notify retailers to not honor checks written on this account. In most cases, the bank is responsible for any losses. To find or check whether someone is passing bad checks in your name, call the Shared Check Authorization Network at (800) 262-7771.	

includes how to protect yourself from identity theft and how to respond if you are a victim of identity theft.

Select Aggressive Antivirus Software

Aggressive antivirus software should be part of your technology plan, not only as an initial purchase but also with annual and periodic updates to ensure that your technology devices are secure. Any time your antivirus software generates a report, log on to view any dangers or threats to your information and computers. Hackers once took pleasure in announcing how they had hacked into secure websites. Today's hacker is much more sophisticated and seeks to fly under the radar for financial gain. Nearly all antivirus software protects you from the following:

- *Spyware:* Software that tracks your online behavior without your knowledge or consent.

- *Adware:* Advertising-based software that displays pop-ups and advertising messages.

- *Keyloggers:* Software that tracks your keystrokes and can be inadvertently installed if you click on a suspicious link.

- *Malware:* Malicious software designed to disable or damage your computer.

- *Rootkits:* Allow a hacker to take total control of your computer at the root or administrative level. Antispyware programs can detect and eliminate rootkits.

- *Trojans:* Malicious programs.

Aggressive antivirus software also guards your technology devices against the following:

- *Phishing:* An attempt to obtain sensitive information, such as passwords and credit card information. These usually are attached in an e-mail.

- *Viruses:* These may be in your removable devices, such as USB drives.

PC Magazine frequently reviews antivirus software and provides reviews. Some of their more highly reviewed software includes the following:

- Kaspersky Anti-Virus

- Bitdefender Anti-Virus

- Norton Symantec

- Sophos

Key Takeaways

In this chapter, you learned the following:

- Everyone needs a technology plan.

- Your technology plan can be used to help manage passwords, financial accounts, and processes you can put in place to protect your accounts.

- Technology has added tremendous value, as it helps to manage much of the information that caregivers must address.

- Technology also comes with cautions, but a good technology plan will make your life much easier to manage.

In section 1, you got through many of the major hurdles of "what do we do now?" Section 2 focuses on tools that will help the caregiver in the day-to-day experiences that help protect loved ones. Cool Tools in section 2 are intended to help you enjoy life while you are tending to a loved one.

Section 2 | DAY-TO-DAY TOOLS

If you are an app geek or if you've ever wanted to delegate tasks to someone else but didn't feel comfortable doing so, you will love this section. This section guides you through a comprehensive review of tools that can be a lifeline for caregivers. Start by putting a good Internet security plan in place to protect you and your family's important information. Then load up on apps that help you coordinate schedules, monitor medications, or create a safe environment for loved ones at home. This section also provides guidance on how to manage medical bills, understanding your rights as a caregiver, and tools for selecting a home for your loved one. Legal and ethical planning is not a solo activity, but we provide tools for you to establish a communication plan so that when you need a plan on short notice, one will be there for you.

05 | Healthy Living Tools and Mobile Apps: Getting You Teched Up

Another day. Your mom is already awake sitting at the breakfast table watching the morning news. The dimmer switch barely sheds light into the room, but you can see the blue glow of the television, and you know her morning routines haven't changed.

But your morning is rich with new possibilities because you have some Cool Tools that will make your caregiving tasks easier to manage her care. You make the kids' lunches and remind your husband of his dentist appointment today. You may even find time to go out with friends tonight after work. It could happen. This chapter focuses on mobile applications, medical devices, and emerging technology designed to make your life as a caregiver a little more fun and certainly more interactive.

According to a 2011 study, Bringing Caregiving into the 21st Century, conducted by the National Alliance for Caregiving and the United Health Group, participants were asked what kind of mobile apps they wanted most (see figure 5.1).

"Make my loved one feel safe and reduce my stress" is what 72 to 77 percent of all respondents said they looked for in helpful tools. "Also, help me feel more effective as a caregiver, manage logistics better, save time." This chapter is here to help.

As caregivers ourselves, we also found that our families maintained multiple lifestyle plans. Caregivers maintain a stringent schedule of medication, meals, and daily diagnostics, such as checking for insulin levels. Sometimes we get so caught up in our own routines that when friends and family offer to help, we say, "Oh, thanks, but I'll do it myself. You just cannot imagine Mom's restrictions." Friends reminded us that this approach limits the caregiver. It suggests that helpers cannot help. "I can do it myself" interfered with our loved one's social needs. So we launched in-depth searches to find healthy living tools—mobile

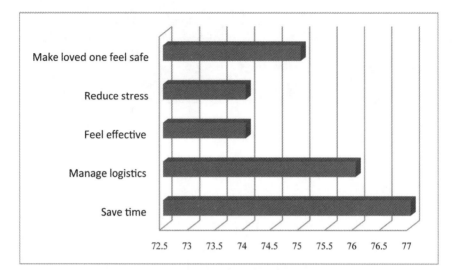

Figure 5.1. What Caregivers Want in Mobile Apps

Results from Bringing Caregiving into the 21st Century reveal what caregivers want mobile apps to do for them.

applications that caregivers can use to inform helpers without appearing to be overprotective or controlling.

Our App Selection Process

Globally, software applications for iPhone, Android, and Windows users, as well as Web-based ones, are launched into the consumer marketplace with lightning speed, making our selection process time sensitive. Their advertising goals to consumers are to help you do the following:

- Become more productive.
- Manage multiple details.
- Share communications.
- Enjoy the experience from using their tools.
- Pay next to nothing for the app.

The business goals don't always align with user goals, but that doesn't mean they aren't well intentioned. Business developers of apps want to see the following:

- Rapid adoption of technology (consumers are happy using the app and will tell others).
- Quick return on investment.

- Real-time operational intelligence, meaning that developers can study how users make decisions. Developer decisions require features such as alerts that require your response to improve the app.

In selecting the apps and healthy living tools for you, we tested them against eight factors:

1. Is the app built from a reliable company?
2. Has it been successfully tested to play well in the iPhone, Android, or Windows environments?
3. Is it secure?
4. Is it affordable?
5. Is it relevant to the caregiver?
6. Does it provide warnings before you destroy important information?
7. Are graphics pleasant to the user?
8. Is it fast?

Security First When Using Mobile Apps

Before downloading apps onto your tablet or smartphone, be sure that your security measures are in place.

- Do not auto-save critical passwords that allow anyone, including a hacker, to access or open your financial apps.

- Password protect your device and, in particular, use a password before making any financial transactions.

- Set up features to find your smartphone or shut down specific features in the event it is stolen or lost. Most likely, your smartphone has confidential information that could identify you.

- Enable your Device Security Manager on your Android or iPhone.

With security measures in place, let's get to the Cool Tools.

Nine Most Important Features in a Mobile App

Ann Napoletan posted a blog on Caregivers.com that listed the nine most important features to look for in caregiver's app. Before you start loading up your smartphone with apps, review these nine features, adapted for you here:

1. *Helpers:* Does the app invite helpers, or trusted friends, to help?
2. *To-do lists:* Does it track to-do lists?

3. *Journal:* Can you keep a journal that allows you to record observations, share photos, and keep family members in the communication loop?
4. *Profile:* Does it let you maintain personal information, such as allergies, insurance information, blood type, Social Security number, and religious preferences, in a single place?
5. *Calendar:* Does it track appointments and send you reminders?
6. *Contact list:* Are family and friends at your fingertips in the event you need help?
7. *Medication tracking:* Does the app help you keep track of meds, dosages, prescription numbers, refill information, and send reminders?
8. *Secure documentation storage:* Does it allow you to upload secure documents, such as advance directives or health power of attorney?
9. *Broadcasting of communications to family members:* We consider this nice to have, but your smartphone likely also has this feature.

Cool Tools: Meal Planning

TakeThemAMeal.com

The next time friends from your faith community, neighbors, or coworkers ask how they can help, direct them to TakeThemAMeal.com, a website inspired by church and support groups devoted to helping members deal with crisis and comfort. Set up your free account before sharing with others or ask a friend to help build an account for you. On this website, you can do the following:

- Register the meals you need.
- Select with whom who you'd like to provide easy directions to your home.
- Select healthy recipes you'd like someone to make for you.
- Select which days you need meals delivered.

Long-distance family members who often seek ways to provide help can visit the site, order a meal that serves from two to twelve people, and have it delivered to your home.

Pushpins

Caregivers often make a dash to the grocery store to pick up an item needed for dinner and end up purchasing additional items that may languish in the refrigerator unused for days. What we liked about Pushpins.com is that it allows the user to begin by selecting a meal. Pop-ups identified ingredients in the grocery store you will need to complete this meal. In addition, the app also links to eBates for current coupons, many with manufacturer bar codes, that you can present at any grocery store's checkout. Even for noncaregivers, this app turned out to save both time and money.

GroceryIQ

When reviewing Grocery IQ.com, we liked the ease of building a list of items that we frequently purchased into a Favorites list simply by checking "+" from the "Favorites" tab. Also, while we were in the "Dairy" section, Grocery IQ pop-ups reminded us of other items on our grocery list within that section so that we could avoid rushing back from the "Bakery" to find something left behind in "Dairy." We could choose frozen foods last.

We used the built-in camera from our smartphone to take a picture of the product's bar code as one way to load up a grocery list. If you prefer, you can bar code items in your home as you run low on supplies. Items are then uploaded into your grocery list. Currently, you must connect with Coupons.com for a digital scan of coupons before checking out, or you can print coupons at home and bring them with you. The app becomes intuitive about your purchasing habits and prompts you with current coupons. This app lets you create and replicate grocery lists via text or voice-based instructions. You can send your grocery list to another smartphone user, such as a spouse, who views anything beyond the magazine rack as a navigational challenge.

Cool Tools: Coordinate Schedules

In the same study, Bringing Caregiving into the 21st Century, 70 percent of caregivers said they wanted an electronic calendar that coordinated doctor's appointments, soccer practices, and business appointments. We found several apps that support caregivers of all ages and cultures. As mobile health expands, more apps will become available. We will continue to list our favorites on www.Caregivers-Toolbox.com.

Cozi.com

Recently acquired by Time, Inc., Cozi.com is a family organizer with more than 10 million users. Cozi won the Mom's Choice Award in 2009 and 2010 and the National Parenting Center Seal of Approval in 2008, 2009, 2010, and 2011, among other awards. This is a free mobile app and website that helps you manage your family's schedule, your loved one's medical appointments, and to-do lists and view individual schedules or the whole family in a color-coded calendar.

Cozi leverages your Google Calendar to get you started. As this is a free app, count on some pop-up ads to track your shopping and appointment schedules. Blog posts were ambivalent about Cozi's acquisition by Time, Inc. However, the giant company promises to offer customers more stringent control over privacy practices.

Personal Caregiver

Seventy percent of family caregivers said they wanted an app or device that reminds the patient about his or her prescription medications. Caregivers who support loved ones taking multiple medications may find that the Personal Caregiver app can be used by the caregiver or by the loved one when the caregiver is away. This free or low-cost for premium subscriptions supports unlimited medications lists and reminders and missed dose alerts and reminds you when refills are due.

Caregivers can also see if the loved one missed a dose. We offer caution when reading the missed dose indicator, whether on this or any other app. A missed dose could mean the following:

- The patient took the medication but didn't turn off the reminder on the smartphone.
- The patient turned off the reminder but didn't take the medication.
- The patient took the medication and turned off the reminder.

Be sure to communicate with your loved one what the reminder means and how to turn off the alert. This may be challenging for loved ones who are vision impaired.

Medication-dispensing services, such as ManageMyPills offered by Philips, costs about $50 per month with a one-time setup fee. You load the medications into the dispenser and program the time for each medication. When loved ones hear the alert at the programmed time, they press the dispenser and take the medication. Connect the dispenser to your phone line if you want to be alerted when your loved one misses a medication prompt.

These apps will help if you are coordinating schedules for one family. Once you coordinate your and your family's schedules, consider building a process for church friends, family, neighbors, and others who want to help into a community.

Apps in the section "Cool Tools: Coordinate Friends and Family into Your Caregiving" (see next page) are the ones we found to be both secure and either free or very low cost.

Caregiver's Touch

The Caregiver's Touch app is for both professional and individual caregivers, but the pricing clearly delineates the two types of users. Essential features include the following:

- A calendar for caregiving events, especially if you are caring for more than one person

- Medication management, including doses and schedules

- Caregiving contact lists

- Medical history logs

The iPhone app costs $4.99 per month, and professional caregivers will want to add the Web-based version for $19.99 per month.

GreatCall.com

GreatCall.com supports the generation of older Americans determined to maintain independence and mobility, the same ones who keep you at the edge of your seat at work, unsure where they are or if they have forgotten their way home. GreatCall offers a small waterproof device with a 5Star Medical Alert button, Splash, for wireless help 24/7. Similar to Onstar for cars, the Splash button connects your senior to a live operator trained to immediately stabilize the caller and then connect the caller to your mobile or home phone. GreatCall's Splash typically is embedded in Jitterbug5, a large-number cell phone and medical alert combination. Splash also may be embedded in smartphones with built-in medical alert features. In an emergency, the Splash and GreatCall's SmartPhone device will connect you to certified emergency dispatchers or to nurses and board-certified doctors for urgent guidance. The MedCoach app embedded in the smartphone sends prescription reminders to keep your loved one on schedule.

The Splash, Jitterbug, and GreatCall smartphones are affordably priced and also require a subscription to a wireless phone network. GreatCall is endorsed by John Walsh, safety advocate and vice chair of the organization. Splash is $49.95, Jitterbug5 with GreatCall inside is $99, and SmartPhone with built-in medical alert apps is $149.

Cool Tools: Coordinate Friends and Family into Your Caregiving

Caregiving is anything but a solo activity. Sometimes the incredible compassion you have for your loved one is so overwhelming that there could never be anyone who delivers care as well as you. Likely that's true.

Let's say your loved one spends up to six hours in chemotherapy, dialysis, or similar treatment. At first, you are the one and only person ever allowed to be at your loved one's side, ensuring that the infusion of drugs is completed accurately and compassionately. After a few weeks of missed work or nights of lost sleep, you may be much more willing to allow friends to help with transportation.

This is when the transition from "Superhuman You" turns to "Fabulous Circle of Friends." You may feel a little shy asking for help at first, but technology can be such a cool door opener. For example, you might say, "Remember when you offered to help? Let me show you this cool tool."

For privacy and potential identity theft reasons, we encourage you to avoid sharing health care requests on unsecure social networking sites, such as Facebook, Twitter, or Instagram. Use an app hosted in a secure environment where you can approve or remove participants.

Tyze

Tyze is more than an application for your smartphone or tablet. It is an interactive network model that brings together multiple relationships into a confidential community that celebrates successes while keeping your loved one safe through a supportive network.

Tyze calls its network a "social convoy" of caregivers that may include the home health provider, immediate and extended family members, family physician, or trusted neighbors. All are driven by the need to support your loved one. Clearly, some are employed, such as the physician and home health worker, but the intent is to bring together medicine and technology to "engage, connect, and inform the individual and their personal network members to co-create the best outcomes."

Created and located in Vancouver, British Columbia, Tyze partners include more than fifty organizations in Canada, the United States, and the United Kingdom as well as the Robert Wood Johnson Foundation, the U.K. Department of Health, and the J. W. McConnell Foundation.

Check out the provoking YouTube discussion on Tyze: how sons and fathers are taking care of their fathers. The point of this discussion is that men often feel awkward talking about how they care for their fathers when, in truth, men are often caregivers for wives, children, and fathers.

CareZone

Earning plenty of attention these days, the CareZone portal connects friends and family into a community that shares caregiving tasks. What sets CareZone apart from others is the development team's sense of humor and personal commitment to caregiving. The CareZone app is currently free but likely will be offered in graduated price ranges: free, extended, and premium. Developers are devoted to industrial privacy as they bring experience from leadership roles in publicly and privately held international companies. We are confident that this app will be stable for the long haul. CareZone is based in Seattle, Washington.

Get Your Loved One Up and Moving

According to the *Journal of Aging and Physical Activity*, range of motion that engages muscle and connective tissues directly impacts quality of life and survivability. Your loved one may fear musculoskeletal injuries if he or she engages in exercise, but if you focus on strength building, stretching, and joint movement, you also improve the immune system. A four-year study on the "epidemic of disability" among adults seventy-five years and older showed that adults are able to live independently and longer when engaged in stooping, bending, kneeling, handling, fingering, and reaching.

We found it more fun for our loved ones if all those activities were wrapped around playful Cool Tools that also engaged other members of the family. The hard truth is that most of the loved ones we care for are not going to be in the Senior Olympics. They will, however, find that strength is the single most important function in their body, helping to manage osteoporosis, arthritis, balance, back problems, type 2 diabetes, obesity, and pulmonary diseases. Ask your physician about any of these Cool Tools, stretches, or weightlifting.

Isometric exercise, once the fad of the 1970s promoted by Charles Atlas, is back in style, especially for seniors. Isometrics involves tensing your muscles without movement. Isometrics don't increase range of motion or flexibility and can increase your blood pressure, which is why we want to be sure your loved one's physician is part of this routine.

Progressive resistance training also strengthens muscles. Use free weights of five pounds or less or elastic exercise bands.

Cool Tools: Physical Movement

ElderGym

ElderGym provides thirty-six videos: twelve each for trunk and back exercises, lower body exercises (ankles, hips, and knees), and upper body exercises (arms, biceps, triceps, and shoulders).

Pocket Yoga

Loved ones looking for a more Zen connection can download Pocket Yoga for $2.99 onto an iPhone, Android, or Windows phone. You also can watch the yoga stretches on television or connect wirelessly through a tablet. Exercises are layered in easy, moderate, or intense for loved ones and their adult children to do together.

Taoist Tai Chi

Taoist Tai Chi for seniors is good for balance, circulation, increased strength, and flexibility, a real benefit for loved ones managing muscular diseases such as muscular dystrophy, people recovering from car accidents, or others trying to maintain flexibility. Seniors may enjoy the gentle turning and stretching movement.

Wii Games

Once considered games for children and families, seniors and individuals trying to maintain or improve range of motion have taken up the art of Wii games to such an extent that Wii now includes long-term care facilities, rehabilitation centers, university exercise facilities, and senior centers. Favorites among seniors include the following:

- Wii Fit

- Wii Sports is one of the less expensive Nintendo games. Tennis and Bowling require low-impact movement. Golf, Baseball, and Boxing focus more on range of motion.

- Big Brain Academy is a Wii game that helps keep the mind sharp and is recommended by the American Association of Retired Persons. Wii Degree is a virtual college that offers puzzles and math problems for players to solve with up to eight people who can participate at the same time.

- Rock Band offers the thrill of performing live music using video game instruments. For seniors who love to sing or for latent rock stars who never made it beyond karaoke on Throw Back Thursday, this is a great game.

Cool Tools: Brain Workouts

KnowTheBible

KnowTheBible is a free application for computers with hundreds of Bible trivia games. Included are Bible passages, daily Bible verses, and Bible study guides. As with all computer games, be sure that your antivirus software is updated. The KnowTheBible website selected Norton Security, and users can click on advertiser links to make purchases.

Lumosity

Lumosity is a scientifically developed network of brain-training games with published studies that demonstrate the effects of using Lumosity on healthy adults, children, cancer survivors, and individuals trying to maintain cognitive skills. Customize your account to select the type of brain challenges you or your loved one want to play. For example, decide how much you want to improve your memory, pay attention to details, increase your speed in response time, engage in problem solving, or increase flexibility, such as quickly adjusting to changing rules. Workouts are approximately fifteen minutes per day.

Once you've set up your account, you can change settings if your loved one has over- or underestimated brain and dexterity capabilities. These games can be done one-on-one or with friends working together in the same room or on a social network, such as Facebook. Games are free during an orientation period and then are available for a fee on a monthly basis. Download Lumosity on any device, including smartphones and mobile devices.

Key Takeaways

In this chapter, you learned the following:

- In seeking technology tools that help, caregivers want tools that do the following:
  - Make my loved one feel safe.
  - Reduce my stress.
  - Help me feel more effective as a caregiver.
  - Help manage logistics better.
  - Find tools that save time.
- Keep security at the top of your mind when downloading apps onto mobile devices, laptops, and home computers.
- Consider Cool Tools that help improve your loved one's range of motion and memory.
- Put safety first when guiding loved ones on how to manage medications.

In chapter 6, we will explore how apps and mobile devices can help you make your home or the home of your loved one a safer place to live.

06 How Technology Can Support Caregivers at Home

Aging at home helps seniors stay at home, but due to the increasing limitations of what seniors can and cannot do, technology can help caregivers, whether they live next door or across the country. This chapter is designed to provide Cool Tools for daily activities that can be used by you or your loved one. These tools also will help bridge the gap between the following:

- Aging-at-home seniors who may never have learned how to program a VCR.
- Caregivers using smartphones, iPads, and apps to stay mobile while caring for loved ones.
- Aging seniors and kids who started using technology before they learned to walk, a great resource for those of us learning how to use new applications or devices.

In this chapter, we provide guidance on the following:

- Home safety checklists you should reference periodically to keep the aging at home or disabled generations safe.
- Home-monitoring technology to alert you when there is a problem.
- Easy-to-use tablets and handheld medical devices that monitor symptoms such as glucose levels, blood pressure, and oxygen levels.
- How telemedicine can help your loved one reach specialists 1,000 miles away without leaving your hometown.
- How virtual office visits can help fill the gap when you aren't sure if your loved one needs to come into the medical office.

Technology: Not the Final Answer; Rather, a Great Lifeline

Caregiving and technology will continue an unprecedented growth as baby boomers take on care for their parents, their spouses, or returning members of the military with special needs. Boomers have long anticipated the freedom to visit their adult children and grandchildren, travel, and enjoy retirement. Many learned technology, and some even invented it along the way, with each following generation expanding its reach into technology. Today's grandparents are relearning technology under the tutelage of three-year-olds to third graders. They also are using smartphones to take pictures of grandchildren or texting to stay in touch. Boomers also use apps that allow them to communicate through virtual cameras, such as with Skype or FaceTime.

Home is where technology can be most useful, and it's also the place most people want to stay if they are still active and managing life skills, such as personal hygiene, mobility and rehabilitation, cooking and eating, housecleaning, and finances. When these essentials are in place, technology is available to help when time is not on your side. Certified "aging in place" specialists, one of the newly designated careers to help support aging adults, is seeing rapid adoption of technology among caregivers and their loved ones. In this chapter, we start with the basics of ensuring a safe place for your families and loved ones.

Start with a Home Checkup

As a caregiver, you may be skilled at managing two or three phones at once, Face-Time with family, or using Skype for long-distance telephone and video. As you dive deeper into technology tools for the home with your loved one to help your loved one accept some technology in the home, we suggest beginning with a safety checklist. A safety checklist does the following:

- Gives you a reason to launch a discussion about technology and home safety.

- Lets you better understand your loved one's anxieties about using technology.

Your ultimate goal is to keep technology tools from getting pitched or used as a doorstop when you aren't around.

> About every three months, my brother Steve and I did an informal inventory of our mom's house to be sure she was equipped with enough support to live on her own. Our inventory was a room-to-room checklist that helped her maintain

her independence but also ensured she could access immediate help if she needed it.

Kitchen

Lighted Large-Digit Phone: We purchased a digital speakerphone with large numbers and programmed our cell phones into her lighted speed dial. We also programmed her grandchildren's phone numbers so that she could stay in touch with them as well. Then we purchased a large-print address book and transferred all entries from three-by-five card files, address books from her insurance agents, and slips of loose paper into the address book.

Check:

Phone:

- Were there unheard messages on the phone?
- Did she need more addresses added to the large print?
- Did power outages affect her speed dials?

Cabinets:

- Were chemicals stored away from foods?
- Were there signs of pests?

Appliances:

- Were appliances still working?
- Had any cords been compromised?

Floor:

- Was there grease on the floor that would cause her to slip?
- Were there any items that could cause her to trip?

Fire safety:

- Does she have a current fire extinguisher?
- Does she know how to use it?
- Are outlets overloaded?

Refrigerator:

- Was there something fuzzy growing on her foods?
- Had the food expired quite a while ago?
- Had the refrigerator been cleaned recently?
- Did it need a service call or new filters?

Low-Vision Tools: Mom had macular degeneration and glaucoma, but she regularly exercised her mind with large-book logic puzzles and large-print books. But her monthly bills didn't come in large print, so she purchased a **Low Vision Smart Reader** for about $2,500. Used ones are available in black and white on

Craig's List and eBay now for $25 to $100. She used her Smart Reader to write bills, balance her checkbook, copy new recipes, or read and hand write letters, a rare gift in today's social networking community.

Check:

- Were there any service contract or maintenance updates?
- Has anything dropped to the floor that would cause her to slip?
- Was she keeping up with bills?

Large-Number Digital Scale: Although her mind hardly declined, other parts were not so cooperative. To help her manage congestive heart failure, her doctor put her on diuretics, but she had to weigh herself twice each day to ensure that fluids weren't accumulating. We purchased a digital talking scale, not something every woman wants within earshot, but she lived alone.

Check:

- Can she still see the scale without tripping over it?
- Does it still work?

Pill Reminders: A child of the Great Depression, Mom was a detailed penny manager, especially when it came to medications. Her theory: take only what you need until you feel better and save the rest for when the doctor won't write a script. We found pill bottles that had expired more than five years previous to her passing in 2010.

Check:

- Is she taking her meds?
- Are some of them cut in half?
- Is she storing unused meds under the bathroom sink?
- Does she know side effects from irregularly taking her meds?
- Is she playing pharmacist with Dad's meds?

Trash:

Check:

- Can she still carry garbage bags out to the garage?
- Can she still wheel trash bins to the street?

Family Room: Mom loved to sit in her La-Z-Boy and watch TV, but she struggled to see the remote. We put small pieces of electrician tape on both sides of the remote and then marked one side V for Volume and the other side C for Channels.

Check:

- Can she get in and out of her chair okay?

- Is the carpet stretched to avoid tripping?
- Is the temperature adequate for her?
- Can she get to the bathrooms without obstacles?

Bedroom:

Check:

- Did she need extra bulbs for her night-lights?
- Was she running low on personal make up?
- Was she doing the laundry?
- Did she need a new toothbrush or mouthwash?
- Was she keeping her weekly hair appointments?

Bathrooms:

- Were the basins draining properly?
- Were toilets flushing without overflowing?
- Were the rubber stops on her shower chair wearing thin?
- Does her handheld showerhead need to be cleaned?

Home Security:

- Did the doors still lock? Are the deadbolts in use?
- How many people have a key, other than family?
- Did the house look lived in? (i.e., grass mowed, leaves periodically removed from back deck and gutters)
- Were neighbors watching out for her? (Each time we were home, we walked over to the neighbors and church friends and thanked them for helping Mom. We also wanted them to know we knew she relied on them.)
- Could she get out of the house in an emergency?
- Were the smoke detectors working?
- How did she handle inclement weather?
  - Did neighbors shovel the walk when it snows or after ice storms?
  - Did she have somewhere to go in the event of high winds?

(Carolyn Hartley)

Cool Tools for Home Checklists

Use our checklist provided in this example and add content as you wish or use checklists at these sites:

- *A Place for Mom:* Use this checklist to help determine if your loved one needs caregiving assistance.

- *Consumer Product Safety Commission:* Choose "Safety for Older Consumers Home Safety Checklist" under the "Safety Guides" section of this site. This is one of our favorite checklists, as it offers great details and is thorough, taking you room to room through the house. The checklist is intended for aging-at-home seniors.

- *National Safety Council:* Checklist to manage falls. Tools on this site offer facts about older adult falls and an older adult fall prevention checklist.

- *Caregiver Home Care Checklist:* Home care safety for the caregiver.

- *Home Safety for Alzheimer's and Dementia Patients:* From the Alzheimer's Association. How Alzheimer's disease and dementia affect safety in the home. A valuable checklist for all elderly care.

- *Homemods Assessment Tool:* From the Fall Protection Center of Excellence. One of the best assessment tools on home safety for the elderly.

Transition into Technology

Soon, pacemakers may be the size of a small pill. A nanosensor implanted in your loved one's finger will trigger a phone call that your loved one is two weeks from a heart attack. Sounds like decades from now, but these tools are already in development for consumers. Take a look at our picks for Cool Tools that help seniors transition into technology.

Cool Tools That Provide Technology Product Reviews for Seniors

- *CAST, Center for Aging and Services Technologies:* Reviews safety technologies for seniors. Enjoy watching a video that demonstrates how current technology can support aging in place with the story of Alma, an eighty-three-year-old woman who goes from home to hospital, rehabilitation, and back home.

- *Aging in Place Technology:* Care.com. Introduces technology to help seniors who wish to remain in the home.

- *Abledata Device Reviews:* From Abledata, an independent source for assistive technology devices in home safety. Provides reviews and directs you to company websites. Products are not marketed or sold on this site.

- *Verizon Wireless:* Provides product reviews of apps that can be accessed on the Verizon network.

- *A Place for Mom:* A really cool agency that acts on your behalf to find a place suitable for loved ones. The company also supports aging at home as long as your loved one is safe.

- *Kaspersky:* One of the most highly recommended antivirus software companies with international labs that monitor emerging threats.

Cool Tools for Vision Impairment

- *The Snapfon:* Created for individuals with vision impairment. Provides cell phones with big buttons, enhanced sounds, and Bluetooth-enabled hearing capacity. An SOS button transforms the phone into an emergency line for seniors.

- *Vtech:* Provides a phone with photos of family members in place for speed dial. A portable pendant serves as a speakerphone for one-touch dialing and can be clipped to a belt.

- *Jitterbug:* A cell phone made with seniors in mind, with one-touch access to health and safety experts. Nice features include easy navigation, big buttons, and a loudspeaker. This is a pay-as-you-go phone service.

- *LGExalt:* A good flip phone for seniors that offers clear sounds and a large three-inch screen for storing pictures or browsing the Web. It's a bit heavier than a smartphone, but the size makes it easier to find in a pocketbook or beside the bed. Call plans are tailored toward seniors. Verizon, for example, offers the phone for $9.99 per month and a two-year agreement.

- *Telikin:* An easy-to-use touch-screen computer for seniors. Easy to view and maneuver. Price is higher than tablet computers.

Cool Tools for Exercise and Mobility

- *WiiFit:* An exercise product to help one build balance while having fun. Requires you to have a Wii system. Balance board is included. WiiFit has become a new staple with assisted living facilities to maintain mobility and promote community.

Cool Tools for Internet Security

- *HTTPS Everywhere:* Protects your loved one from hackers lurking in WiFi hot spots, keeping the Internet safe for loved ones wanting to stay in touch via e-mail with family and friends while the caregivers are away at work.

Webcam Etiquette: Useful for You and Your Loved One

As a caregiver, you recognize and accept that you cannot monitor every step your loved one takes while alone in the home. Webcams can be a useful tool for caregivers when a loved one is living in the home alone, but a valid concern is how to balance the use of webcams with your loved one's privacy.

We offer key points to consider before putting webcams in the home:

- Receive permission from your loved one to allow a camera to be installed, as trust and respect is the foundation for being a caregiver. Caregivers sometimes try to justify with their loved ones that "the webcam is only to monitor you in case you are alone and fall again." If this is true, the caregiver should check to see if there are medical issues, such as osteoporosis or orthostatic hypotension, that would require an alternative living arrangement. Understanding the true reason for a webcam will build trust and respect.

- Receive permission from your loved one for camera location or locations. Yes, the bathroom and shower are key areas for accidents with the elderly, but perhaps the camera should be in the living room or outside the bathroom. Dignity has its place.

- As a caregiver, especially if you are a family member, you sometimes think a camera may be the best solution for watching your loved one if he or she is alone in the home. It helps remove the worry about your loved one's safety but also raises the question, "If you are so concerned for your loved one, should he or she really be left alone?"

- In the event that another person is helping with your loved one's care, we recommend that you inform him or her of any cameras installed in the home.

Cool Tools for Web Monitoring

- *Lorex:* A wireless home video monitoring system that can be easily installed in your loved one's home and configured to monitor multiple rooms. Remote monitoring is accessed by logging in to the home camera via your iPhone or Android. Available for $199.

- *Vuezone:* A remote video monitoring system used to stay in contact with your loved one. Each system is battery operated with wireless cameras that can be installed in any room with "peel-and-stick" magnetic mounts. Remote monitoring is accessed by using your iPhone or Android smartphone. Price ranges from $129 to $229.

■ *Grandcare:* Gives caregivers the ability to remotely monitor loved ones who are living in their own homes. Buyer will have to purchase Grandcare's hardware and software, depending on the level of service provided.

Medication Management

Medication management can be one of the most difficult and tiring areas a caregiver must deal with.

My dad took thirteen medicines each day, while my mom, who was doing her best to assist him, took seven daily medications for her own health. This is not uncommon. It took a lot of concentration each week to keep their medications sorted properly while double-checking correct dosage amounts.

Many people also try to self-medicate (treat themselves without medical supervision) due to the financial burden caused by having a large number of prescribed medications. Early in my career, I was employed as a pharmaceutical representative for a top cardiovascular medication. A concern of the cardiologists and other physicians I called on was the high price of our medication, which was causing some patients to change their prescribed doses. For example, instead of taking two pills each day as prescribed, some patients were self-managing their medications by breaking pills in half or taking only once per day in an attempt to lower their costs.

(Peter Wong)

"Almost 30 percent of all hospital admissions for people over the age of 65 are directly attributable to medication non-compliance," says Andy Schoonover, chief executive officer of VRI, a health care services company with twenty years of experience in remote monitoring, medical management, and medical alert systems.

How can the caregiver meet this challenge and manage medications for his or her loved one who wishes to stay in the home? How can one ensure that proper doses are taken at the correct time? Is there a way the loved one can self-manage prescribed medications with or without the caregiver's help?

Technology innovations in medication management have gone beyond the basic plastic pillbox. There are now medicine-dispenser tracking tools available that deliver correct medication doses, have alarm reminders, and lock for safety. A National Institute on Aging study of the benefits of electronic pill dispensers found that using these dispensers cut the number of days people forgot to maintain their drug regimen in half. It also improved their ability to remember to take a second or third dose of their medicine.

Cool Tools for Medication Management

- *E-Pill Station:* Medication management to assist your loved one with taking medications. Locked dispenser with alarms. Suggested retail price $450. No monthly fee.

- *Pocket Pharmacist:* Prescription pocket pharmacist app for iPhone and iPad. $0.99. Provides drug information and interactions for patients. Also a medication organizer. It is like having a pharmacist with you.

- *MedReady Pill Dispenser:* Medication management to assist your loved one with taking medications. Locked dispenser with alarms. Medical alert monitoring, medication adherence, and vital sign monitoring services can be added. Price varies by services ordered and range from $30 to $50 per month. Price includes monitoring service.

- *Medication Dispensing Service:* Medication management to assist your loved one with taking medications. Locked dispenser with alarms. Medical alert monitoring, medication adherence, and monitoring system can be added. There is a one-time installation fee of $99, with service options starting at $49 per month.

- *MedMinder:* A pill dispenser with built-in cellular connection; no need for Internet or phone line. Locked or unlocked dispenser available. Price varies by services ordered and range from $39.99 to $64.99 per month.

Cool Tools for Monitoring Vital Signs

Some tools help the caregiver with administrative burdens. For example, the caregiver may be taking vital signs of his or her loved one each day and recording the information for a future doctor visit. Rather than recording statistics in a notebook manually, technology makes it possible to record the information using a smartphone or tablet. Blood pressure, oxygen levels, heart rate, and blood sugars are examples of vital signs that can be measured and sent to your physician. Talk to your doctor about how to exchange information electronically. Your doctor's office can suggest ways to send vitals to the patient portal. Patterns and discrepancies in your loved one's condition can be assessed by your doctor, allowing him or her to determine the next course of action without the loved one's leaving the home.

Cool Tools for Blood Pressure Monitoring

- Most of the blood pressure monitoring and glucose reader tools advertise that you can send data directly to your physician. That feature depends on whether your physician's patient portal can take updates from your smartphone or tablet. Sending content into your portal does not guarantee that your physician will review the findings, but during your visit, you and the physician can open your portal account to review findings (if the practice allows this).

- *Medisana BP Monitoring:* Medisana CardioDock 2BP and Monitor, iPhone and Android enabled. Blood pressure recording and monitoring. Can be used to send posted data to your physician. Not approved by the Food and Drug Administration (FDA).

- *Smart BP Monitor:* Withings Smart BP Monitor, Apple devices enabled. Blood pressure recording and monitoring. Can be used to send posted data to your physician. FDA approved.

- *iBP Blood Pressure App for iPhone:* Easy to use and send posted data to your physician. $0.99. Smart BP Monitoring device is required.

- *iBP Blood Pressure App for Android:* Easy to use and send posted data to your physician. $0.99. Smart BP Monitoring device is required.

Cool Tools for Glucose Monitoring

All glucose monitoring devices sold in the United States must be FDA approved. Some glucose devices that do not bear the FDA approval signs have resulted in false readings, resulting in serious injury or death. While we offer some of our favorite monitoring systems, there are many others with FDA approval. An app for iPhone or Android adds value and convenience for you and your loved one:

- *OneTouchVerioSync System:* A glucose meter that can send sugar readings to your Apple device. Uses OneTouch Reveal mobile app for Apple devices. $29.99. Test strips not included. FDA approved.

- *iBGStar:* iBGStar Diabetes Manager blood glucose meter can be used independently or with an app for iPhone and Android. The iBGStar blood glucose measurement and monitoring system, when integrated with an app, shows you instant results and also provides trend lines. Ask your physician if their patient portal accepts results from this app. The application can be purchased online or at some drugstores. $71.99 to $74.99. FDA approved.

Apps That Connect Glucose Meters with Smartphones

- *OneTouch Reveal App:* One Touch Reveal Blood Sugar Monitor app for iPhone or Android monitors blood sugars. The app is a companion to the OneTouch glucose meter. Test readings can be sent to your physician, but you will need to check with your physician to see if readings can be uploaded to the patient portal. To be used with the OneTouchVerioSync System. Free.

- *BGluMon:* App for iPhone and iPad that can send sugar readings to your Apple device. Easy reporting features. $3.99.

Cool Tools for Heart Rate and Oxygen Levels Monitoring

- *Cardiobuddy:* Touch-free heart rate monitor for iPhone. Seen on *Dr. Oz.* Fun to use. Free. After a few initial uses, the app will transition into a low-cost monthly subscription.

- *iSPO2:* Masimo iSPO2 Pulse Oximeter for iPhone and iPad. Measures heart rate, respiratory rate, and blood oxygen levels. $249.

- *Zensorium-tinke:* Tinke's Pulse Oximeter app for iPhone and iPad. Measures heart rate, respiratory rate, and blood oxygen levels with Bluetooth option. Free app. Tinke device required.

  - *Tinke Device for Android:* Tinke Oximeter for Android. $129.

  - *Tinke Device for iPhone:* Tinke Oximeter for iPhone. $109.

- *iHealth-SPO2:* iHealth Wireless Pulse Oximeter app for iPhone and iPad. Measures and tracks blood oxygen levels and heart rate. Free.

Stepping out of the home and into the medical office can be a daily or a weekly occurrence, and that is where technology is advancing. Telemedicine and its companion, virtual office visits, connect you with physicians when timing and travel stand in the way.

Telemedicine/Virtual Office Visits

Your loved one has mobility difficulty, or you have five hours left this month for personal time off from work, and a trip to visit a specialist in San Diego is not in your budget or your schedule. Wouldn't it be nice to see the specialist without having to leave your hometown?

With advances in telemedicine, home health visits, virtual office visits, and mobile applications, you can sit with a nurse practitioner at a local hospital or in an eight-by-five kiosk and be examined by doctor in another city, another state, or another country. It may sound like something from *Star Trek*, but advances in technology like these will continue to improve and enhance our ability to be better caregivers for our loved ones.

Telemedicine is the use of modern telecommunications technology between patients, providers, and their support teams to exchange medical information. Patients and physicians connect via videoconference using computers, tablets, or smartphones rather than in a traditional office visit setting. This is one of a variety of virtual office visits taking shape across America.

If asked to describe why telemedicine is gaining momentum so quickly, the answer would be convenience. Currently used in remote areas, telemedicine allows patients and their caregivers to go to a smaller critical access hospital and sit with a nurse practitioner who collaborates with a physician 100 to 2,000 miles away to diagnose, treat, or prescribe a care plan providing quality care. With the advent of newer technology and a push from the Affordable Care Act, telemedicine can provide patients with better care, lower costs, and greater access to advanced care regardless of age, illness, or geography.

A telemedicine appointment would look something like this: You or your physician's office obtains preauthorization (approval) that your insurance company will pay for telemedicine services. Most insurance companies will reimburse for this consultation.

You may be asked to wear a monitoring device for a few days prior to the visit so that the specialist can view trends, such as when you experience irregular heartbeats or glucose changes during the day and night. Some of these devices will have a smartphone app attached so that you also can view the trends. Telemedicine can also be used for mental health visits, so you may be asked to maintain a diary prior to the visit.

Your physician will schedule an appointment at a hospital or clinic that has telemedicine equipment in place. Telemedicine centers must demonstrate that they are secure, preventing any unauthorized access through their network.

When you arrive for the appointment, you will be brought into a room with a video camera, a computer, and an exam table. Sitting with you in the room is either the physician or a nurse practitioner. You will be introduced to a specialist on the computer monitor who is in either another city or another country, but your physician trusts his or her judgment to help solve your problem. The specialist will ask the clinician to provide results from your monitoring device or perform a physical exam and report the findings back to the specialist.

If the specialist recommends a procedure, he or she will guide the clinician through the process, but first you will be made comfortable, for example, with a local anesthesia to relieve any pain. Procedures are typically scheduled at a different time and place so that you are treated in a sterile environment. You check out as you would a normal office or hospital visit, and your provider files a claim on your behalf for payment.

Sound interesting? Telemedicine can certainly save you time and money. To find out if telemedicine services would work for you, begin with a conversation with your provider. As of 2015, forty-eight states provided some form of Medicare or Medicaid reimbursement for telemedicine services, and some private insurers have expanded their coverage of telemedicine for mental health and high-risk stroke care. Look through our telemedicine directories to help in your search.

Some of the health practice specialty areas that may currently use telemedicine technology include cancer and blood diseases, cardiology, dermatology, nephrology, pediatric telecardiology, and many more.

The Cincinnati Children's Hospital in Cincinnati, Ohio, for example, offers eConsults to children and their families around the country. This service is provided via e-mail, video, and phone and gives access to children's physicians specializing in rare diseases who can review your case and collaborate with your local doctor.

Another example is the Cleveland Clinic's launch of a "Virtual Visit" telemedicine trial with Time Warner Business Class in 2013. By providing health care services to remote patients, this trial highlighted the benefit of savings both in the time needed to see physicians and specialists and in costs to the health care system and patients. In most cases, telemedicine reduced the burden of patient travel and costs.

Virtual Office Visit (Retail Health Clinics)

Virtual clinics are being established in nontraditional health care settings, including large businesses and retail locations with clinics. Some hospital emergency departments also are jumping into the business.

Rite Aid and Wal-Mart are examples of telemedicine-based retail service virtual clinic locations, with CVS, Walgreens, and others likely adding virtual clinics in the future. A virtual clinic visit may have a shorter wait time and cost less than a trip to your primary care physician.

A virtual office visit is similar to a telemedicine appointment, with a few differences. In a virtual office visit, you connect online directly with a health care professional for a fee that you pay by credit or debit card up front. The fee will range from $49 to $99, depending on the service and time you need with the provider. Virtual office visits generally do not include a clinician at your side, but you will be communicating directly with a professional.

Several high-volume stores, such as Target and Wal-Mart, offer virtual office visits. To see how one works, go to the Web, use the search words "Wal-Mart's

Virtual Clinic," and watch a YouTube video that describes how you can participate in a virtual clinic visit.

Cool Tools for a Virtual Office Visit

- *Teladoc:* The first and largest telehealth provider in the United States, serving over 7.5 million members, is a 24/7/365 service for nonemergency medical issues or short-term prescriptions and a convenience for caregivers when loved ones cannot make it to your primary care physician. To use this service, contact Teledoc by phone or online and set up an account to become a member. Complete a questionnaire using information typically provided in a new patient visit. You may then schedule your visit, either a phone or online video consultation with the doctor. Teledoc says that the average response back from their board-certified physicians is sixteen minutes, and your consultation with the doctor has no set time limit. In the event you need a specialist, Teledoc can advise you on whom you need to see. Their website also offers a video to walk you through the process. Teledoc can issue a prescription for antibiotics, antihistamines, and other short maintenance medicines that comply with your state's regulations. Teledoc cannot issue prescriptions for controlled substances, such as antidepressants, or for nontherapeutic drugs, such as Viagra or Cialis. Teledoc's costs may be reimbursable, but first check with your insurance plan or employer to see if they are in the Teledoc network. Teledoc can also check their database to validate this information for you. Teledoc members pay a $9.95 out-of-pocket fee per month, and each consultation is $40 out of pocket if your insurance plan or employer does not provide coverage for Teledoc services. Teledoc is not meant to replace your primary care physician.

A growing trend among midsize and larger physician practices is to offer their own virtual office visits. In this scenario, you would communicate with your own provider through the webcam built in to your computer. Examples of providers whose existing patients can communicate virtually with them are included here.

- *Healthspot:* Integrates telemedicine and virtual medical visits into a single location. "The key," says Lisa Maughan, HealthSpot's vice president of marketing, "is not only to give consumers easy access to healthcare services, but to also offer providers an opportunity to connect with patients—both their own and potential new ones—when and where they need healthcare. These visits also pull people out of waiting rooms, enable quicker care for conditions that don't require a face-to-face visit and free up doctors' time to focus on the more acute cases."

- *Telehealth Kiosks:* In mid-2014, insurance company Kaiser Permanente teamed with the Cleveland Clinic to introduce virtual clinics called telehealth kiosks. The kiosks offer consumers a private videoconference with a doctor and include access to diagnostic tools and electronic medical records.

- *Mercy:* The sixth-largest Catholic health care system in the United States, Mercy began construction on the country's first virtual care center in mid-2014. "Telemedicine lets us provide the best possible care to people where and when they need it—even when patients wouldn't otherwise have access to specialists, such as neurologists and pediatric cardiologists," says Lynn Britton, Mercy's president and chief executive officer. "The center will bring together the nation's best telehealth professionals to reach more patients, develop more telemedicine services and improve how we deliver virtual care through education and innovation."

Key Takeaways

In this chapter, you learned the following:

- Advances in technology are changing the way caregivers can support loved ones in the home.

- There are many home safety–based apps you can access with your computer or smartphone to support you as a caregiver.

- Webcams can play a role in helping the caregiver but must be balanced with your loved one's need for privacy in the home.

- Caregivers should take advantage of the flexibility and convenience that virtual office visits, virtual clinics, and telemedicine can provide.

07

Manage Medical Bills

Physicians know that you may love and trust them for the care they bring to you and your family, but when the medical bills start pouring in, the love–trust relationship gets a bit shaky. When medical bills exceed 5 percent of income, consumers are twice as likely to have trouble making ends meet. Pulling out a credit card to pay for the hospital or physician fees is not the answer. In this chapter, we offer details on how health care professionals get paid and what you can do to navigate successfully through that process.

The Health Care Billing Process

When you purchase a house, the seller posts a price and negotiates what you will pay. Your real estate agent carries the terms of the agreement back and forth. You may want to purchase the furniture, appliances, and draperies currently in the home, and the agent negotiates these numbers on your behalf. To ensure that the house meets local quality standards, you hire a mechanical inspector. You pay the broker and the agent a commission for working on your behalf. Health care billing processes are nothing like this.

When you purchase a car, the dealer recommends a price. You look up the car's value in the Kelley Blue Book or NADA's Guides and shop around to learn what other dealers charge for the same car. Some of us take the car to a mechanic to see if the car meets quality standards. You even have three days to bring it back if you aren't satisfied with the results.

But when it comes to health care, neither the health care professional nor the patient knows the real cost of the service. That's about to change. When consumers started purchasing high-deductible insurance, they finally had an opportunity to discover what other providers charge for the same service and still receive the same or better quality

Figure 7.1.   Medical Billing Processes and You

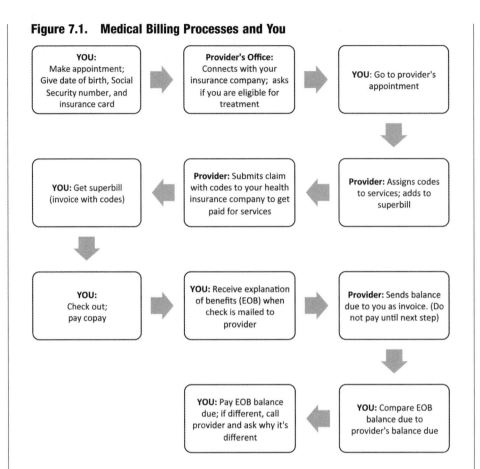

of care. But first consumers needed access to data other than the patient's copay and the deductible. Consumers also needed to understand the language, which is mostly in code.

Until 2014, health care billing and reimbursement processes were clouded by clinical language, billing codes, bundled services, and negotiations where you were not invited to participate. Even so, you were still expected to pay your part.

Let's dig in and demystify health care, starting with key definitions. We've highlighted definitions that will translate into your secret weapons to better understand your bill. These definitions are intentionally not in alphabetic order. Instead, they replicate the billing and medical costs process (see table 7.1).

Key Definitions

Beneficiary: In health care insurance terms, the beneficiary is the person who has signed up for, qualifies, and pays for health insurance benefits.

Eligibility: Eligibility means that, according to the plan you selected, your health insurance determines for what service you are eligible to receive benefits.

For example, when you call to make an appointment, the scheduler asks for key information. The provider can determine your eligibility using three pieces of data (information):

- Your date of birth
- Your first and last name and correct spelling
- Your insurance plan subscriber number

These three pieces of information are used to instantly verify that you have insurance, what kind of insurance you have for hospital stays (major medical, or Medicare Part A), physician services (preventive health, persistent health issues, or seasonal illnesses—Medicare Part B), and prescriptions (prescription coverage, or Medicare Part D). For our techie friends, this is the HIPAA 270/271 transaction. This information may not be released to anyone except the provider, supplier, or beneficiary.

Secret Weapon #1

Superbill: This is a form that contains an itemized list of services that health care professionals use to describe the reason for your visit and the treatment or procedures you received. This form is the backbone for how the provider gets paid. Your doctor must sign a copy of your superbill as you leave the exam room or hospital and hand it to you for checkout. Each practice customizes its own superbill according to several factors:

- The types of patient visits they are most likely to see.
- The types of procedures they are most likely to perform. This may include injections, laboratory orders, skin scrapings for biopsy, stitches, and so on.
- The superbill is the practice's list of services they offer, except there aren't any prices associated with the fee, only codes and the physician's signature.

Prior to the Affordable Care Act ("Obamacare"), consumers did not pay as much attention to the superbill because their costs seemed to be limited to copay and a small deductible. In today's higher-deductible environment, be sure to save the superbill, as it is the key to managing your fees. *Checkout:* Most health care organizations request that you make your copay before you see the doctor or receive treatment. Remember that they did an eligibility check before you came into the clinic, so they have a pretty good idea of what you owe. Sometimes the cost is more than you can pay at one time. Health care organizations typically understand this and will work out a payment program for you. We cover that process in this chapter.

Secret Weapon #2

Billing codes: Billing codes are just that: numbers or a series of numbers and letters that are used to describe to the insurance company details about the health care you received. In a physician practice or urgent care facility, there are several types of codes, but the two you want to know are these:

- ICD (International Classification of Diseases), version 9 or 10
- CPT (Current Procedural Terminology).
    1. *ICD codes:* The International Classification of Diseases (ICD) codes identify your disease. In the United States, there are between 33,000 and 75,000 ICD codes, depending on which version (ICD-9 or ICD-10) the Centers for Medicare and Medicaid Services (CMS) requires your doctor to use. Pneumonia, for example is a disease, and there are about 250 ICD-9 codes for various types of pneumonia. Coders hired by the organization look at the physician's notes to help determine which code to apply for billing.
    2. To treat pneumonia, the doctor creates a plan that may include a procedure. Your health care provider is reimbursed for also documenting the procedures using a Current Procedural Terminology (CPT) code. A few procedures for pneumonia might be the following:
        a. Oxygen or antibiotics for viral pneumonia
        b. A complete blood test to check white blood cells
        c. A CT scan of the chest to see how the lungs are doing

To get reimbursed, the ICD (diagnostic) and CPT (procedure) must align. For example, the provider shouldn't order a brain MRI for a woman who complains of a cough unless the woman also complained of severe headaches. There are many more complex codes that hospitals use, and we will use some Cool Tools to explain those.

Secret Weapon #3

Explanation of benefits: Within a day or a few days after your visit to the health care professional or hospital, the organization will submit a claim on your behalf to receive reimbursement. You will receive two documents:

- An invoice from the doctor/hospital showing your balance due.
- An explanation of benefits (EOB) showing you what the insurance paid and what you owe the provider. The amount you owe the provider is based on a contract the provider has with the health plan that essentially says,

"If you plan to accept our insurance for our customer's health care, you, Mr. Provider, cannot charge more than XXX amount, and the organization will need to write off the rest." The amount you owe is based on that agreement. Remember that although this is one of your secret weapons, you may not agree with the amount you owe.

Do *not* pay the invoice until you receive the EOB.

How to Read Your EOB

Your explanation of benefits is not a bill, but it is one of the secret weapons you need when managing your health care costs. An EOB is generated and mailed to you the day after your insurance company paid the provider. Your EOB is required to tell you three important things:

1. *Summary of charges.*
   This is a summary of the bills your health care provider is asking your insurance plan to pay.
2. *Plan accumulations.*
   This section shows you how much money you have paid to date for out-of-pocket health care services. This amount also shows how much remains until you meet your annual deductible.
3. *Claim detail.*
   Table 7.1 provides a chart and companion description of what a claims detail looks like and what it means. Information provided here is fictitious to avoid exposing anyone's confidential health information. Let's say your loved one went to the doctor's office complaining of heart palpitations and anxiety. The physician ordered a blood test.
   In table 7.1, note the clues in bold that will help you understand what the insurance company paid, what the insurance company required the health care professional to write off, and what you are responsible to pay.

Do you see the hidden fees you've already paid? Your insurance said you owe a $20 copay and another $20 to the provider. But the checkout clerk collected $30, so you are already $10 ahead of what you owe. Your invoice from the doctor should be $11.60.

Let's Manage Your Medical Costs

Between 45 and 100 percent of the time, your medical bills are inaccurate. With two decades of experience in health care, I assume that they have an error 100

Table 7.1. Your Explanation of Benefits (EOB) and What Each Column Means to You

Type of Service	Submitted Charges	Plan Allowance	Remark Codes	Deduct	Coinsurance or Copay	Medicare or Other Insurance	What We Paid	What You Owe
Therapeutic care	120.00	97.48	610	0.00	20.00		77.48	$20.00
Diagnostic pathology	37.00	10.68	610		1.60	0.00	9.08	1.60
ICD and CPT codes are embedded here, but you cannot see them. They were on your **superbill**.	These are the providers' fees. Every provider has a fee schedule, but they rarely publish it. (See section on self-pay.)	This is the amount your health plan allows to be billed according to the provider/ plan contract. The contract was completed before you stepped into the clinic.	This remark code (610) means that the provider's fees exceeded your plan.	This is the amount applied to your annual deductible. Your annual deductible may be on page 2 of your EOB.	This is what the insurance says is your copay. But wait, in this case, you paid $30.00 (copay) because that's what the checkout clerk requested. You've already paid $10 more against your invoice.	This is what was billed to your secondary insurance and what they paid. In this case, there is no secondary insurance.	This is what your health plan paid the provider.	This is in addition to your copay. The amount here should match your invoice.

percent of the time, the same approach I take when hiring an attorney, a plumber, an automotive repair service, a consulting subcontractor, or a builder. The Medical Billing Advocates of America, Consumer Reports, Elderweb, and Medical Bill Rehab indicate that the current error rate is between 70 and 85 percent and even up to 90 percent for the elderly. Stephen Parente, professor of health finance at the University of Minnesota, said in a *Wall Street Journal* article that he estimates that errors might be between 30 and 40 percent. In the same article, Joe Fifer, vice president of hospital finance for Spectrum Health in Michigan, says that he demystifies costs by offering estimates up front so that patients know the cost before entering the hospital.

Even if the ratio of incorrect codes is one to three, these numbers can be pretty alarming. The Commonwealth Fund, a nonprofit organization that focuses on health care research, says that credit scores from medical billing errors affect 14 million Americans. Payer–provider contracts are negotiated in such a way that you don't know the real cost of health care. But this chapter is all about helping you become your own medical bill advocate.

Whether you like or dislike the Affordable Care Act, one positive outcome is that health care costs are much more transparent. Given the percentages, chances are pretty good that your medical bills are inaccurate. This isn't an indictment against the physicians or their office staff. You are the person responsible for paying your health care bill, but the process is so convoluted that we trust our providers to file on our behalf.

> My clients who are large health insurance companies also agree that there is confusion in the marketplace, and with the implementation of the Affordable Care Act, consumers should pay close attention to their medical bills. Some of their senior management admitted to me that while caring for their loved ones, they found errors in their own medical bills. They recommended that the consumer always check and validate them.
> (Peter Wong)

When health care providers file your claim, many people and computerized software programs get involved in the process. Here we provide some sleuthing techniques and Cool Tools to help you manage your medical bills. It helps to separate the billing process from the relationship you have with your doctor. Your doctor provides care, but the doctor's team manages the invoices.

To begin your discovery process, pull together three documents:

- Superbill

- EOB

- Invoice from the provider or hospital

Step 1: Begin with the superbill .

You probably received a yellow and a pink copy of your carbonless bill when you left the practice. Hospital invoices may be printed documents, but they have a similar structure. This document is called a superbill because there is so much data (information) embedded that the provider will use to file a claim for reimbursement. It also is your receipt for charges you paid.

This form puts the claim process in motion, so look for some of the following more common errors:

1. Procedures: Did the provider indicate you had a procedure done?
    a. A procedure is something the doctor did for you during your office visit or hospital stay. This could be an injection, a skin scraping for a biopsy, or a spirometry (test for asthma), or it could be more complex, such as a colonoscopy.
    b. Check to be sure there is a CPT code next to the procedure. You may need to compare prices that other providers charge. We'll show you how to compare prices in our Cool Tools section.
    c. Did you need preauthorization for those procedures? Your health insurance will likely pay for medical procedures completed in the practice, but some require a prior authorization. This means that you or the practice must get the insurance company to clinically review your medical situation before approving the procedure. For example, a doctor may want to inject Botox into your knee to relieve joint pain, but the insurance says, "No, first get tested for nerve damage. If your care team determines there is no joint damage, then go back and get an injection." Doctors today also must prove that some tests and procedures are "medically necessary." If you bypass the payer's preauthorization and get the Botox injection first, the doctor's claim will likely be denied, and you will be billed the full charges. The injection may or may not work, but without a preauthorization, you pay whether it worked or not, according to your insurance plan's details.
    d. If during checkout or discharge from a hospital you are asked, "Do you want a charge summary or an expanded invoice?," always ask for the

expanded invoice, especially if you are concerned about the costs that will be charged.

2. Your superbill also is your receipt for what you paid.

3. Be sure the superbill is signed by the physician, indicating that changes won't be added without your knowledge. Physicians rarely add to the superbill without a good reason that also includes a call explaining those charges to you.

Step 2: Let's go to the EOB.

1. Does the type of service match what actually happened? Did you come in for an office visit, or did you come in just to see the nurse for a tuberculosis test?

2. Do you understand the types of services? If not, call the practice and ask for clarification on the medical term. Diagnostic pathology, for example, is more complex to understand than "blood test," but the physician may get reimbursed more if it's called "diagnostic pathology."

3. Check out the difference between the submitted charges and the plan allowance. Submitted charges are always higher. If you have high-deductible health insurance, you certainly want to know who is negotiating this down on your behalf. If that's your case, we will provide you with Cool Tools in the next section.

4. Most important, look at what you owe the provider. This number may not agree with the provider's invoice, especially the case in table 7.1, where you paid $10 more in copay than what was required.

Step 3: Compare your invoice with your EOB and the superbill.

1. What does the invoice say you owe?

   a. In the example provided in table 7.1, the invoice should be for $11.60, not $21.60, as the EOB suggests.

   b. That's because you overpaid your copay by $10.

2. Was your doctor in network but you were billed at out-of-network rates?

   a. In network means that the payer and provider have a contract that says that the provider agrees to receive payment from this payer at a prenegotiated rate.

   b. Out of network means that you will pay higher percentage of fees because the payer and provider did not have a contractual agreement. Your payer will still reimburse the doctor the same as an in-network provider, but since your payer has not negotiated your rate, you pay more. Sometimes people choose to pay the higher fee for second opinions or to see a surgeon with more experience. Often you can negotiate an in-network rate with the out-of-network provider.

c. When you scheduled your first appointment with the doctor or hospital, the scheduler should ask, "Do you have insurance?" Depending on your answer, the scheduler should also tell you whether the provider accepts (in network) or does not accept (out of network) this payer.

3. Were you charged for lab work?

    a. The lab test should be circled on your superbill.

        i. Some lab work is gender specific. For example, a man should not be charged for a Pap smear.

        ii. Were you charged several times for the same test?

    b. Did you ask how much the charges will be? Very few people ask and then are surprised when they receive a lab invoice from an outside company.

4. Were you charged for a brand-name prescription and then given the generic?

What If the EOB, Superbill, and Invoice Don't Match?

If the numbers don't line up and you cannot figure out the discrepancy, take heart. You won't be the first, and you sure won't be the last to make some calls. Most people call the insurance company to get answers.

We like to call the organization that submitted the bill first. This could be the medical practice, rehab center, or hospital. Call and ask for the billing department. Most likely, you will get routed to the people who assigned codes to your visit. Remember that it's the codes that insurance companies reference to pay the doctors. Medical coders, usually very well trained professionals, can answer your billing question.

Start by saying, "I'm trying to understand my invoice, can you help?" Medical coders and billers often are on the front lines of angry patients and caregivers who don't understand the medical terminology, let alone the costs, so it can put everyone into a tense situation. Take a deep breath and remind yourself that you are seeking clarity, not confrontation.

Describe the situation. For example, "It looks like my mother is being charged for an EKG, but I was in the office with her getting medication for her sore throat. I don't recall her ever getting hooked up to an EKG monitor."

Coders cannot change a billing code without the physician's approval. Physicians aren't going to change a billing code to accommodate patients who cannot pay for the visit. However, the physician will correct an error if during the visit you mentioned something that would change your clinical documentation. That change may mean changes to what your insurance will cover and the final amount you owe.

I disputed a $1,072 medical charge for more than two years and made a commitment not to give up even after my charges were sent to two collection agencies.

My nurse practitioner, under the direction of a doctor I never saw, recommended I get an injection of Reclast, a drug used for patients with osteoporosis. I had been taking oral medications for several years for mild osteopenia, and the adult nurse practitioner said I would be a good candidate for Reclast. Today's protocol for my osteopenia is to take over-the-counter calcium, but Reclast was new, and osteoporosis was high on direct-to-consumer television advertising. I also would learn more as the collection process heated up.

In previous years, I sat with my brother and sister during their cancer treatments, so I did not take infusions lightly. I began my research on side effects and costs by logging on to several blogs to read results from other consumers on this injection.

Then I looked up the drug's billing code for a "Reclast Injection (J3488)." I searched the medical literature and billing resources on the average cost of an injection. At the time, infusion costs ran from $750 to $1,500, depending on location. The facility would also charge a fee for administering the drug. I then called our insurance carrier, asked how much they would reimburse, and learned it would be about 80 percent. Note: I've changed from using the term "injection" to "infusion." "Injection" to a coder means less than fifteen minutes. "Infusion" means more than fifteen minutes, and Reclast takes about sixteen to seventeen minutes (i.e., higher billing).

All went well until I got the EOB. The infusion center charged my insurance carrier more than $7,000. I was in shock when the EOB indicated that I would owe the provider $1,072. I called the doctor's office and said, "Stop all referrals to this clinic because their invoices are completely out of range."

I called my insurance carrier and filed a formal complaint that the infusion center charged such exorbitant costs when it was completely out of range. Our carrier filed a complaint on my behalf with the infusion center, which responded that the charges were "within contract limits." I asked to see the contract. My health insurance company denied my request. I also filed my complaint with the employer, who said, "Take this up with the insurance company."

Dissatisfied with being caught in the middle, I dug deeper into the Novartis website, as they were the pharmaceutical giant producing Reclast, and found the approved billing codes for outpatient infusions. J3488 was the code for practices and hospital-owned infusion centers for the drug, but 0636 was the code to be used for administering inpatient only infusions. My bill was coded as if I had been an inpatient: 0636.

I called Novartis's help desk to be sure I was tracking the right billing code. The Novartis help desk said the price was one of the highest he'd ever heard of nationwide, but there was nothing they could do to help. He did confirm that the correct code for outpatient infusion was J3488 but that the infusion center could charge their normal fee to administer the drug, about $400.

Imagine my surprise when I called the infusion center's billing department and my call was transferred to the hospital's billing supervisor. His response was that I should have gone to a different facility where fees weren't as high. Really? I wrote down his comment, along with his name, phone number, and time of our conversation, as I was certain his supervisor would be thrilled to know his customer service strategy: "If you don't like our costs, you should have gone elsewhere." Short of throwing the phone at the wall, I recalled my training and asked for a detailed cost summary of my encounter. I would need evidence to get through the finger-pointing.

When the hospital's detailed invoice arrived, I wrote a response disputing the charges, citing the discrepancy in billing codes, and attached my full billing summary, noting that nowhere was the J3488 code. A month later, another set of invoices came, and I disputed those charges in writing as well. Five months went by without a call, an invoice, or a letter. Then I received a letter from a collection agency accusing me of ignoring any of the hospital's attempts to collect. Attached to the collection agency's invoice was a one-page summary of my hospital charges. Sure enough, there it was, 0636, with no reference to J3488.

Before responding to the collection agency, I began making more phone calls and dug up as much information as possible. This is what I learned:

- The infusion center had been purchased by a hospital system a few weeks before my infusion.

- The practice that had referred me to the infusion center now also was using the same tax ID. All of them were in on this referral. This means that revenue came to the practice that referred me for treatment. That is a potential violation against the Stark Law.

- The hospital filed my claim not using the former infusion center's tax ID but now under the hospital's tax ID, which meant significant upcharges.

- I went to the Centers for Medicare and Medicaid Services (CMS) and looked up the prices they paid for treatments. While I wasn't on Medicare or Medicaid, I also knew that CMS set a standard for other payers to follow. Reclast Injection was among those published costs.

I pulled my findings together into a large envelope and sent copies of my findings, including my notes from the billing administrator's conversation, to the collection agency.

About one month later, the collection agency sent me a letter saying they would no longer contact me about these charges and apologized for any convenience.

But then a year later, the collection agency was purchased by a larger collection agency. Agency 2 sent me a letter that they had purchased Agency 1's debt and intended to collect $1,072 plus 14 percent interest on the unpaid balance.

I prayed, "Come Holy Spirit. Show me what to do." I was one person against a large hospital system who could out-finance my legal fees any day. At the time, there were no medical advocacy groups to take on my case. To the hospital, I was just another patient with a debt problem. But I had done my research, and I knew they had used the wrong codes.

I sent Agency 2 a letter along with copies of my previous correspondence, along with the letter from Agency 1 that the account was closed.

Agency 2 responded with a letter that they intended to collect.

I let the letter sit for a few days in my Bible. Tucked in such a safe place, I hoped some guidance would pour into my bill.

At wits' end, I filed a complaint with the state's attorney general citing a collection agency's attempt to collect on the hospital's inaccurate coding. I also stuffed the envelope full of copies of my evidence.

I did not hear from Agency 2 for a long time. But after thirty days, I received a letter from the state's attorney general. The attorney general's letter said they had investigated the matter and included a written response from the new billing supervisor. For the first time, I saw the billing code, J3488, in my invoice, the very code that had not been in any of my previous documentation. Had the hospital doctored the code for the attorney general? Or had I missed something in my research? After a few weeks of hearing nothing, I called Agency 2 and asked about the status of the claim.

"We have a cease and desist on your account, ma'am. I'm not allowed to talk to you."

"What does that mean?"

"That means I'm not allowed to take any action against you. The hospital has dropped charges."

On the one hand, I was deeply relieved. Regardless of whether I had won, the case was closed. My regret, however, was that the hospital, according to the terms of its insurance contract, still made $5,000 more than an infusion center would have billed for this treatment.

I wish my story was not so common, but in telling it to the new breed of medical billing advocates, I've come to respect their due diligence on behalf of patients. Their response to me? "That's nothing. Let me tell you my story."

(Carolyn Hartley)

The New Breed of Medical Billing Advocates

The Affordable Care Act has given birth to a new industry of medical debt defenders who will take on your case for a fee if you believe that your medical charges are out of range. Sometimes their fee is a percentage of the debt they can recover for you, or their fee may be an outright daily charge. Medical billing coding for hospitals and physician practices is a rapid-growth area for education and training, largely to support billing and coding for both consumers and health care professionals. Wise and experienced coders make for great medical bill defenders.

Cool Tools

If you need help from a medical bill defender, consider reaching out to these organizations:

- *American Association of Professional Coders:* Many of its members achieve licensing credentials that we look for when speaking with a coder. In looking for assistance, be sure the person defending your debt is a licensed coder. This may include the following:

  Certified professional coder (CPC)

  Certified coding associate (CCA)

  Certified coding specialist–physician based (CCS-P)

- *Medical Bill Defenders:* This is a firm of medical billers and coders who can help you evaluate your bills to determine if they are accurate. This group offers free consultation and medical bill review.

- *HealthAdvocate.com:* This group works typically with employees encouraging providers to lower medical bills. The group uses industry pricing data and pricing trends to negotiate costs.

- *Alliance of Claims Assistance Professionals (https://cakehealth.com):* This group provides services including challenging claims denials, negotiating with providers on patient balances, and tracking claims to ensure that they are accurately coded, among many other services. Click on Find a CAP to connect with a professional in your state.

- *VersaClaim:* This group supports employers, patients, and attorneys to appeal claims on denied insurance claims, negotiate claims, and negotiate claims before you go into the hospital.

What If You Are Self-Insured or Carry a High-Deductible Health Plan?

Today, high-deductible health plans mean that consumers are making not only financial choices but also potentially life-altering choices.

- A mother says, "We have another $6,000 in deductibles before our major medical kicks in. The kids come first. We know what their pediatrician charges for an office visit."

- A father says, "Do I really need this back surgery? I will need four weeks to recover, and we can't afford the lost wages. Maybe I can stay on pain medication until I get a better job with better insurance coverage."

- A grandmother says, "I'll be eligible for Medicare in two years. That's when I'll schedule the hysterectomy."

- A father says, "We cannot afford both my epidural injections and our daughter's braces. She deserves a chance I never had, so we will go with the braces."

- A mother says, "I know the cancer has returned. But I don't want to burden my family with worry over my health or costs, so I just won't tell anyone."

The more we know about how consumers are approaching health care and its costs, the better we can provide meaningful quality care that meets their value system. This means a radical shift in how health care professionals share the costs of care. Change won't be easy, but consumers are learning the hidden costs of their health care through several websites and negotiating an up-front fee based on pricing trends in their area.

This trend is one of the most exciting for consumers who, for very good reason, do not want to pay the marked-up retail cost for medical services. Consumers with high-deductible plans should never be asked to pay the same price offered to insurance companies, yet that's exactly what happens. Find out first what the *real* costs are. These are the negotiated-down, real-time payments that insurers pay to cover the cost of their beneficiaries' care. Nearly all Blue Cross Blue Shield organizations offer a cost comparison tool on their state's website.

Cool Tools

Most of the following tools are built on data from the Centers for Medicare and Medicaid Services:

- *Data.CMS.gov:* Here, CMS posts information that would take up more than 44,000 lines in an Excel spreadsheet. To make this easier to read, several companies built software that rides on top of these spreadsheets so that you can more easily access information using their apps.

- *OpsCost:* At this site, you can compare charges for common procedures at over 3,300 hospitals. Select your city, then select the procedure to see what CMS reimbursed for the procedure. The real beauty in using this tool is that you can find actual hospital charges. Website access is free. Once you are on the site, key in your ZIP code and the type of upcoming surgery to find a list of nearby surgical facilities, information about the doctor, and possible complications for the type of surgery or procedure needed. For example, I looked up the cost of a nerve block in my ZIP code and found three locations within four miles of my home, billing an average of $1,098 for the injection. That's the retail price. However, CMS reimbursed an average of $168, or the wholesale price actually paid to this provider. And $168 was the average among all providers in the area. As a consumer carrying only catastrophic insurance, you can take these data to your health care provider and offer to pay out of pocket for the injection. Benefits to you include the following:

  - Much lower cost from your trusted provider

  Benefits to the hospital include the following:

  - Savings from paying staff to file the claim
  - Savings by getting up front and on-time payment
  - Better relationship with patient and family

- *NerdWallet:* This website gathers information about multiple industries, such as banking, mortgage rates, and insurance, and its health component functions similarly to OpsCost. A few additional features we liked were the following:

  - Current feature articles guiding you through additional questions to ask

  - A question-and-answer forum to ask about costs and how to manage bills

  - Links to health insurance exchanges and benefits packages

Cool Tools for Shopping Health Care Costs

- *MyEasyBook:* At this site, UnitedHealthcare supports consumers, employers, and providers by posting prices and encouraging visitors to make an appointment with a provider and then pay for the services through this portal.

- *Healthcare Bluebook:* The Healthcare Bluebook, updated annually, is a guide to help you receive fair prices in your area for health care services. Search by hospital or by physician. You also can search for the cost of a test and consumer reviews on the quality of services. Free online.

- *PokITDok:* This health care marketplace that lets you shop costs and also provides a site for physicians to bid on your care. We aren't so sure that physicians are quite ready to bid on your health care, but it does indicate where health care pricing might be heading.

- *HealthSparq:* This tool provides out-of-pocket estimates based on each member's plan benefits. You enter the procedure, and HealthSparq provides you with costs of services provided at nearby inpatient and outpatient facilities.

- *iTriageHealth:* This is an iPhone/Android app also presented in chapter 3. Using iTriageHealth, you enter your ZIP code and insurance plan, and iTriageHealth analyzes your out-of-pocket costs.

Cool Tools for Employers

- *Castlight:* This is one of the biggest price transparency companies. Customers include Kraft Foods Group, Life Technologies, Honeywell, CVS Caremark, Comcast, and Liberty Mutual. It is available through large organizations so that employers can reduce costs. Prescription drug information is also available for comparison for employers subscribing to Castlight.

Key Takeaways

In this chapter, you learned the following:

- Do not assume that your medical bills are accurate. Do your homework.

- Your three resources to manage your bills are (1) the superbill, (2) billing codes on the superbill that describe your diagnosis (ICD) and procedures (CPT), and (3) the EOB.

- Ask your physician or hospital what the costs will be before agreeing to the service.

- Compare prices and quality of service. Ask a physician or hospital about their success rates if you cannot find them online.

08 | Know the Laws That Support You as a Caregiver

Caregivers are much more than the medication manager, bath giver, family communicator, and financial planner. They are also the patient advocate. Sometimes the patient advocate role can be minimized by health care professionals who appear to dismiss your role, most likely trying to do the best they can for the patient. Other caregivers before you may not have set a golden example of how to be a positive patient advocate. Your responsibilities as caregiver include balancing your rights with the rights also provided to your loved one and to the health care professional.

Content in this chapter is meant to be "just in time." This means that you may want to skip ahead, but at the point you or your loved one's privacy is put into question, the content here will bring its greatest value.

Every patient has a right to expect that his or her health information will be kept confidential and secure, whether providers talk about your situation, write about your case, or share details electronically. Sometimes those rights are overstated and used to keep caregivers at arm's length. If you believe that clinicians have spoken disrespectfully about your loved one or if you have received notice that your loved one's medical or financial identity has been compromised by a health care clinician or organization, this chapter is for you.

In this chapter, we explain the privacy laws that support consumers, patients, and caregivers. These include the following:

- Health Insurance Portability and Accountability Act of 1996 (HIPAA)
- Family Medical Leave Act

Why You Must Know Your Rights

If medical errors were a disease, it would be the number three killer in the United States, third only to heart disease and cancer. In testimony presented to the U.S. Senate in July 2014, Bernie Sanders (I–VT) joined Ashish Jha, MD, professor of health policy and management at the Harvard School of Public Health, in reporting that the number of deaths was so staggeringly large that medical errors took the lives of 1,000 patients per day.

Caregivers often feel put aside by health care providers when they ask safety-facing questions, such as "Did you change your gloves before inserting that IV into my mom?" or "Can we double-check the cancer diagnosis for a possible false reading before you remove my mom's breast?" Today's providers want the caregiver at the patient's side, but administrators have, for good reason, historically feared potential lawsuits, complaints, and audits if the family became too investigative during treatment or a procedure. Practice and hospital administrators use the HIPAA Privacy Rule as an excuse to prevent caregivers from being at the patient's side. There are justifiable reasons to protect a patient's privacy, and those are well defined in the law. But if you are concerned about your loved one's safety, you should exercise your right as a caregiver to be in the room as long as your presence does not compromise the privacy of another patient.

Patients need an advocate to listen and take notes if your loved one is groggy from medication or feels fragile or anxious about a procedure. Get in the middle of the care delivery process and exercise your rights. That's what this chapter is about. Together, we may be able to reduce the 400,000 deaths each year from medical errors.

Health Insurance Portability and Accountability Act of 1996 (HIPAA)

Speak the word "HIPAA" to a health care professional, and watch their eyes roll or listen to them groan. HIPAA is a combination of many rules.

The first part, Portability, was created during President Bill Clinton's first term of office to ensure that you could carry your health insurance from one employer to another without losing your right to insurance. Portability has expanded into an enormously large rule. We won't address that part in this chapter.

The Accountability section also has many laws embedded inside, but the one rule you need to know is the HIPAA Privacy Rule. The HIPAA Privacy Rule applies to personal and medical information about you in written, verbal, or electronic form. You have already experienced part of HIPAA when you or your loved one signed an acknowledgment that you received a notice of privacy practices (NPP). Like most patients, you signed your name indicating that you had received and read the NPP (which, most likely, you did not read or receive), handed the acknowledgment back to the front desk, and sat in the waiting room until the nurse called you back into an exam room. We hope you will never do that again. You aren't giving away any rights whether you sign or don't sign, but neither are you aware of how the practice has agreed to use and disclose your health information.

To understand how HIPAA protects you, take a look at some of the terms used in this rule. We modified the definitions so that they are understandable, but for legal definitions, you should check with a health law attorney or the Office for Civil Rights (OCR), an agency within the U.S. Department of Health and Human Services that protects consumers by enforcing HIPAA's Privacy and Security Rules. Definitions are intentionally not in alphabetic order because each builds on the previous definition. Step with us into the new secret language of HIPAA.

Key HIPAA Terms

Protected health information (PHI): This is personal information about you, such as your name, address, ZIP code, date of birth, diagnosis, treatment plan, medications, lab results, the type of insurance you carry, your insurance copay, your outstanding medical balance, and much more. PHI is what every doctor needs to make medical decisions and get paid for giving you and your loved one treatment and care.

 You expect your PHI to be protected. Someone whom you did not authorize to access your records can cause considerable financial harm to you or your loved one. A few examples of unauthorized access include the following:

- Someone steals a physician's unsecured computer and captures insurance information and your identity to help a family member obtain very expensive drugs, chemotherapy, or dialysis.

- A nosy neighbor may want to know how your loved one is doing. Instead of asking you, the neighbor asks the office receptionist, "We are so worried about Mrs. Jones. Will she get better soon?"

- You may want to pay out of pocket for a service and keep the details of that service from your health insurance provider. For example, you don't want your insurance company to know about a lab test that you suspect the company may use to increase your premiums or to deny coverage.

The NPP is the doctor's or hospital's promise that their organization will safely use and disclose your PHI.

Use: This means that the nurses and doctors on your care team may create your medical chart and add PHI to it each time you come into the practice.

Physicians may access your medical chart from an electronic device, such as a secure laptop or secure smartphone. Each person in the hospital or practice is allowed to see some of your record, but because of their job, most workers will not be able to see all of the chart. "Use" also means that authorized members of your provider team can add details, such as your health care vital signs and medications; document your care; and talk about it among the medical care team. You want the care team to talk about you in a confidential environment so that they can take good care of you. "Use" typically refers to how your health information is managed "inside the practice" or "inside the hospital."

Disclose: In HIPAA, this means to share or exchange your PHI outside the practice to provide treatment and get paid for your care. By law, your PHI may be disclosed for treatment, payment, and health care operations without your consent. Some of the organizations that your physician, urgent care facility, or hospital may share PHI with include the following:

- Insurance companies

- The practice's or hospital's billing service company

- Specialists

- Hospital

- Skilled nursing facility (nursing home)

- Home health agencies

- Physical therapist

- Diagnostic center, such as for mammograms, X-rays, and sonograms

- Collections agencies (for unpaid charges only that are tied to a bill but with no medical details)

Your medical team is not allowed to share details about your or your loved one's care in an elevator or in the hallway where other patients can hear.

Covered entities: A covered entity is a person or organization that must adhere to HIPAA rules, such as the following:

- *Health care professionals:* These include doctors, hospitals, rehabilitation centers, surgical centers, clinics, psychologists, dentists, chiropractors, nursing homes, and pharmacies, among others, that use ICD or CPT codes to electronically bill for services.

- *Health plans:* This includes public (Medicare, Medicaid, military, veterans' health care), commercial insurance companies (Blue Cross Blue

Shield, AETNA, and Cigna), health maintenance organizations, and companies that are self-insured.

- *Clearinghouses:* Most consumers don't know about clearinghouses. These are the companies that process charges for health care clients.

Consent: There are two types of consent:

- *Consent to treatment:* This means that you agree to a medical procedure or surgery. This may also mean that as a caregiver, you agree that the medical team can provide care to your loved one who cannot "act on his or her own behalf." Your loved one may be unconscious, a minor child, or an older adult who is unable to make a clear decision, such as a family member with Alzheimer's disease. For nonemergency care, you may need a legal document called a *health care power of attorney* if you are consenting to a medical procedure for your parents or a family member over eighteen years of age.

- *Consent to disclose information:* This includes consent to disclose information for treatment, payment, and health care operations. According to HIPAA, your health care provider is not required to obtain your consent for some purposes, such as to submit your medical bills to your insurance plan or send medical information to a specialist. However, many physician offices ask that you sign a consent form putting you on notice that the practice or hospital will file medical charges for reimbursement but that you are responsible for your part of the bill, according to your insurance plan.

Authorization: Your health care provider will ask you to sign an authorization form for any activity not included in treatment, payment, or health care operations. Authorizations typically cover the disclosure of PHI not protected by HIPAA's Privacy Rule. Some examples are the following:

- You (the patient) authorize the practice to speak to a family member whom you name about your care. State and federal spouse and child abuse laws may hold the practice accountable if information is provided to the wrong person. As the caregiver, you want your loved one to sign this authorization.

- Your loved one agrees to participate in a clinical trial.

- The hospital wants to send you marketing material to help raise funds for its foundation.

- A pharmaceutical company has asked the doctor to provide a list of patients who would benefit from their drug.

Breach: A breach is an impermissible use or disclosure under the Privacy Rule that compromises the security or privacy of PHI. Nearly all health care organizations have breaches. Some are small and self-contained, while larger breaches make headlines. Of importance to you and your loved one is how they manage the breach internally before your PHI is exposed to someone who should not have accessed it. Considerable civil penalties may occur if a breach is not properly managed.

Privacy official: Each covered entity must appoint a privacy official who oversees and manages the organization's privacy activities. The NPP is required to provide a contact number for reaching their privacy official. Organizations would much rather have you file a complaint with their privacy official than file a complaint with the OCR.

Personal representative: As the caregiver, you may be the person who stands in the shoes of the patient to ensure that his or her rights are protected. HIPAA protects your right to make a health care decision on behalf of your loved one if your loved one chooses to do so. Patient rights also filter to you if you are the legally designated person to make decisions. All states require a *health care durable power of attorney.* Make copies of this and give it to each health care provider involved in your loved one's care. Make an electronic copy for yourself and keep it in your smartphone or tablet for ready access.

Why HIPAA?

You've heard experts in health care say that "the health care system in America is broken." As authors, we hold decades of personal and professional case studies supporting major organizations as they tried to unravel health care's complexity and inefficiencies. The good news is that many organizations are continuing their diligence as the industry faces a $4.7 trillion burden for American citizens by 2020. HIPAA's wide-sweeping changes began in the mid-1990s while Ronald Reagan was president of the United States and Louis W. Sullivan, MD, was Secretary of Health and Human Services.

Many of the nation's health care leaders met in Washington, D.C., to say, "We cannot agree on how to simplify health care and reduce health care costs. You (the federal government) need to force us with standards and regulations." Health care industry leaders, patient advocacy groups, Congress, and federal government leaders jointly created many components of HIPAA, including the Administrative Simplification Act. This act is a set of rules that govern how health care will reduce costs and complexity by transitioning into a standardized electronic environment.

Among President Reagan's and Secretary Sullivan's requirements were that if the framers of HIPAA were to use federal funds to simplify health care and administrative processes, they also must empower all consumers with patient rights. Today, these rights are stronger than they have been in a decade. They allow consumers, caregivers, and families not only to serve as watchdogs for how their PHI is used and disclosed but also to get engaged as active participants managing their health.

Let's look at your HIPAA privacy rights that have been yours since 2003. These should be identified in the NPP that you receive from your health plan, physician, optometrist, dentist, hospital, or any other provider who electronically submits a request for payment for your health services. You don't have to know whether they bill electronically. These are all HIPAA-covered entities.

You received a copy of the NPP the first time you registered with a new provider. You were asked to sign an acknowledgment that you received the NPP, but in many cases, you really did not receive it. It may have been posted on the provider's website or in the waiting room. The point is that by not asking for a copy of this NPP, you bypassed an opportunity to learn how your provider will *use* and *disclose* your protected health information. You did not give up any of your rights, but what follows are the rights that you have that you may not know about.

Here's the short list. In the next section, we provide examples of how to use this right. The OCR also has a cool YouTube about your rights:

1. *Access:* You have the right to access your medical records.
2. *Amend:* If you find something incorrect in your medical record, you have the right to request that it be amended/corrected.
3. *Accounting of disclosures:* You have a right to ask who has seen your medical chart.
4. *Confidential communications:* You have the right to be contacted at one telephone number rather than another or at one address rather than another.
5. *Request restrictions:* You have a right to restrict who can access your PHI under some conditions.
6. *Right to protect your DNA:* If you decide to learn whether a disease is in your genes, your insurance company cannot use the results to make decisions about your coverage, such as increasing your premiums or denying coverage.
7. *Right to file a complaint:* If you believe your privacy or the security of your PHI has been seen or used by an unauthorized person, you can file a

complaint with the U.S. Secretary of Health and Human Services (HHS). By law, HHS is required to investigate.

Want to know more? Let's dig in:

1. *Access:* You have the right to access your medical records.

    How to use this right:

    Begin by asking to see your medical record. Be specific: "I am taking my mother to Florida for the winter, and I need a copy of her medical chart for her physician" or "I'd like to see my father's last five lab results."

    Let's say your insurance carriers have denied a claim. In this case, you can say, "I'd like to receive a patient summary of my mother's visit on <date> and the charges that were applied."

    Caregivers ask for a copy of the chart with much greater frequency than do patients, primarily because they are the caregivers. If the practice is using electronic charts, they will give you a clinical summary each time you bring your loved one into the practice. In a hospital, this is called the discharge summary.

    If the practice or hospital is still using paper charts, they have up to thirty days to pull the chart and provide a summary for you. If the practice is using electronic charts, they can print off a copy within a few days, but as of 2014, HIPAA still allows thirty days to respond to your request.

    The organization has the right to charge you a reasonable fee. "Reasonable" tends to be up to $25.

    The practice may ask you to complete an access request form. That is to help them maintain their required HIPAA documentation.

    If the practice is using an electronic medical chart, they also have a patient portal that you can access, generally at no charge. The organization can set up your own user ID and password to access clinical summaries of your loved one's chart.

    Your request to access medical records may be *denied* for the following reasons:

    ■ You want to see your father's psychotherapy notes. Psychotherapy notes are protected and kept separate from your dad's medical and billing records.

    ■ The provider believes that access to specific portions of your record may cause emotional harm.

- A court document, such as a divorce decree, does not give you access to a child's record.

- The physician believes that the patient for whom you offer care is being mistreated or abused.

You can appeal the denial, but you may need a health law attorney to plead your case.

2. *Amend:* You have the right to be sure that information in your medical record is correct, and, if not, you may request that it be corrected. The key word is "request."

How to use this right:

This right is the most misunderstood of all patient rights.

To amend a medical record means to correct something that is inaccurate. For example, your mother's medical record indicates that she needed surgery on her right shoulder when she actually needed surgery on her left shoulder.

When you request that your record be corrected, you will be asked to identify what is incorrect and how you want it corrected. Your request does not mean the medical practice or hospital will change your record, but if you can demonstrate that the current information is incorrect, HIPAA requires the doctor or hospital to make the change in your record and also to notify any agencies or organizations that received the incorrect information from the provider. If the provider still does not agree to make a change, you can file a statement of disagreement that must be included in your medical record.

How you cannot use this right:

The provider can deny your request to amend for several reasons:

- You ask the billing office to change a billing code to reduce your out-of-pocket expenses. It's possible that the billing code is inaccurate because the record doesn't show something that you and the doctor discussed during your visit. In that case, bring your handwritten notes to the person who manages the practice (practice manager). The physician ultimately must make the decision to change a billing code. However, changing a billing code to reduce your costs could get your doctor arrested for fraud, so be careful about your request.

- You fear that the results of a lab test will increase your insurance premiums and want them changed.

- You don't want your insurance company to know about your most recent diagnosis and ask the doctor to change the diagnosis: fraud again.

- Your preemployment drug test came back positive for an illegal drug. You really need this job, promise to never be a drug user again, and ask the doctor to change the results.

3. *Accounting of disclosures:* An accounting of disclosures means that you want to know where your medical chart has been sent and who has seen your chart. Caregivers who work in health care organizations use this right more frequently than consumers because they want to know who has accessed their medical chart or a parent's medical chart. Accounting of disclosures may be requested by family members managing a loved one with a mental health disorder. For example, your mother has Alzheimer's disease or your father is in a substance abuse or addiction program. You want to protect their privacy and also want to know if anyone is accessing their records who should not be viewing confidential details.

   Accounting of disclosures is a frequent tool of celebrity lawyers protecting their client's identity. Hospital employees peeking into records of George Clooney, Britney Spears, Tom Cruise, Maria Shriver, and Kim Kardashian, to name a few, were fired from their jobs for accessing the chart without permission. The hospital also paid heavy fines and was put on probation for their nosy employees.

   An audit feature built in to the electronic medical record tracks who was in the chart, what they looked at, and if they made any changes to your chart. HIPAA's Privacy Rule and its sister, the HIPAA Security Rule, impose significant financial penalties and possible jail time if an unauthorized person accesses a medical chart.

   An electronic accounting of disclosures may not be easy to read if it is printed directly from the computer. Be sure to request the disclosures in human readable format.

4. *Confidential communications:* You have the right to be contacted at one telephone number rather another or at one address rather than another.

   How to use this right:

   You may have a reason for not wanting anyone in your family to know you have been to the doctor, or you are not yet ready to tell your family about blood tests or mammogram results. Women who may be struggling with spouse abuse are particularly vulnerable. To maintain confidential communications, tell the doctor or nurse that you want health information provided at only one number or one address.

   You will be asked to sign a form that indicates how you want to be contacted. Caregivers must be cautious in exercising this right.

When my father entered a long-term care facility, I held health care durable power of attorney for him because my mother was legally blind. Mom was a brilliant and highly educated woman, but she could not see the flicker on her telephone if someone left a message. Mom and I signed confidential communications documents with the nursing home that they were not to leave a message on her phone. If Mom couldn't be reached, they were to contact me on my cell phone.

An oversight on my part was that Mom's and Dad's friends from the Baptist church knew my toll-free number, which routed to my home phone. The nursing home's nurse supervisor was also a church member and kept calling my toll-free number any time something happened. The toll-free number landed on my home office number, not my cell phone.

At the same time, I was traveling 80 percent of the time helping physicians migrate into electronic health records. Several times, my husband or I would come home from business trips and find an urgent message from the nurse that my father had fallen or was refusing to eat. Each time, I would call the nursing home, stabilize Dad's condition, and plead with the nurse supervisor to always use my cell number. As requested, I refaxed my health care durable power of attorney form, circling my cell number as contact. Finally, I conceded to the nursing home's processes. For patient safety reasons, I opted for a new service that would forward my home phone to my cell phone.

(Carolyn Hartley)

5. *Request restrictions:* You have a right to restrict who can access your PHI under some conditions.

How to use this right:

This is one of the rights that gained teeth in the HIPAA Omnibus Rule of 2013, but it still is a very complex process for a larger practice or hospital to manage. You would use this right for some of the following reasons:

- Your loved one is in a hospital, and you don't want the operator to give out his or her room number. Most hospital policies assume that it is okay to provide callers with the room number. If you exercise this right, you will "opt out" of the hospital's directory.

- You agree to pay for health care services out of pocket and don't want information about that treatment to be sent to your insurance carrier. Make this request with your doctor or hospital.

- You don't want the health plan subscriber (the person who pays health care premiums) to learn details about treatment or a procedure. This is usually exercised by abused spouses.

- You want your prescriptions handwritten rather than sent electronically to one pharmacy so that you can shop for the best prices.

- Your neighbor works at the hospital or practice, and you don't want the neighbor to have access to your loved one's medical record. Unless this person is part of your professional care team, they should not be accessing your loved one's record anyway, but a request to restrict puts the hospital on notice to watch for a possible breach.

To exercise this right, you will be asked to complete a request for restriction of use and disclosure. When completing this form, you must be specific about what information you want restricted. The practice or hospital does not have to agree to your request. If they do agree, they must follow through on your request.

You may not restrict the following:

- A health care professional's right to maintain psychotherapy notes

- Access to medical information in the event of an emergency

A request for restrictions takes time to filter through the staff. Unless the restriction is urgent, be patient until everyone gets on board with your request. However, if time is of the essence, be sure to convey that message to the organization's privacy official.

6. *Right to protect your DNA:* If you decide to learn whether a disease is in your genes, your insurance company cannot use the results to modify your insurance plan.

When a loved one becomes ill, the rest of the family often wants to know, "Is this heredity?" "Could this disease happen to me?" Genomic scientists are building an exciting new world for treating disabling diseases. DNA testing enables doctors to use the patient's DNA as part of the healing process. This is the future of health care treatment, and to keep it safe for consumers, the Food and Drug Administration (FDA) warns that DNA testing purchased by consumers must first achieve FDA approval. HIPAA protects your right to consult a physician for a DNA study without fear that your health insurance carrier will use the results to boost your premiums or deny coverage.

7. *Right to file a complaint:* If you believe that your privacy or the security of your PHI has been seen or used by an unauthorized person, you can file a complaint with the Secretary of HHS. By law, HHS is required to investigate.

How to use this right:

You may believe that your privacy has been breached or exposed to someone who should not have access to the information. It's also possible that the breach could do some harm to you. Some examples are the following:

■ A coworker accessed health information about your loved one and used it as an excuse to block your promotion.

■ A potential employer accessed your health information from your health plan without your permission, and you can prove that the employer used it to deny offering you a job.

■ Visitors to a hospital or medical practice overheard members of the medical team talk about your loved one's condition.

■ A physician or dentist lost a portable tablet that contained PHI, and the practice believes that your medical chart was one on that device. You receive a letter telling you to sign up for a free credit-monitoring service provided by the practice. Be sure you sign up for this service. The letter will also show you how to file a complaint if you think the covered entity is not acting responsibly on your behalf.

If you believe confidential information about you or your loved one has been exposed without your written approval, you have a right to file a complaint with the covered entity and also with the OCR.

You may find that you get the best and fastest response by asking for the physician's or hospital's privacy official. Go to any employee and say, "Something isn't right. I need to speak with your privacy official." A well-trained staff member will ask you to step over to a quiet place and say, "Can you tell me what's happened?" That same staff member will also take notes about your complaint and ask you to fill out a HIPAA complaint form. A smart practice will deal with the privacy issue immediately and also get back to you by phone or letter within days, letting you know in general terms how they are handling this privacy breach. That may be enough for you.

If you feel you are not getting the response you need from the practice, you also have the right to file a complaint with the OCR. You cannot use HIPAA to sue a health care professional, but you can ask the OCR to stand in your defense. No provider likes hearing from the OCR. This agency is required by law to follow up on every complaint and make a decision about next steps. Their decision process determines next steps. Some examples are the following:

- Yes, this is a HIPAA violation. The OCR then notifies the practice that a complaint has been filed and requests documentation to support their version of what happened.

- Yes, this is a HIPAA violation, and you need to get the Department of Justice involved. The OCR also may refer your complaint to another agency, such as the Federal Bureau of Investigation (FBI).

- No, this is not a HIPAA violation. The OCR then sends you a notice thanking you for your concern, but the issue is not a violation.

- No, this is not a HIPAA violation, but it may be a concern for another government investigation. In this case, the OCR will forward your complaint to another federal agency.

The covered entity may not retaliate against you or deny treatment to your or your loved one for filing a HIPAA complaint. You may be entitled to a portion of any penalties the OCR assesses on the covered entity, but you will need a health law attorney to help you determine any damages.

I offer the following story as an example of when to use your right to complain and also as an encouragement to use your rights when you believe something isn't right. This was in 2012, so quite a few things have changed.

My husband is highly successful in his career, and he also has dyslexia, meaning that he often confuses letters and numbers, especially when he is in a high-anxiety situation. I read every document to him before he signs it. When he was scheduled for a medical procedure, I came to the outpatient surgical center with him. He doesn't respond well to Propofol, the anesthesia of choice for this procedure. While a normal person responds to 100 milligrams, my husband has been given up to 300 milligrams.

Prior to our scheduled appointment, we completed his presurgical documentation together, noting the NPP that the surgicenter had us verify twice, once for the online registration and again when we checked in. As explained in the practice's notice, family and caregivers would be called back into the prep room, but friends would have to remain in the waiting room.

While waiting for his name to be called, I noticed that following each procedure, the family member was not asked to come back to visit with the doctor. Rather, the family member was greeted at the exit door by a nurse who went through postsurgical care instructions at the same time the groggy patient was trying to get into the car. All kinds of red lights went off—patient safety at the top of my list.

When the nurse called my husband's name, I stood to go with him into the prep room, but the nurse blocked me, saying, "You can't come back here. It's against our HIPAA privacy policies." I wrote books on HIPAA, and I knew better. That's when my response just spilled out.

"That's not HIPAA, that's your own policies."

"Okay, it's our policy," the nurse responded. "But you still can't come back here."

Stunned, I sat down for a moment not sure whether to make a scene or gather my thoughts. I said a quick prayer for the nurse, another for the anesthetist, and a pretty long one for my husband. Then I left to get a cup of coffee and settle down.

While sitting in the car, I heard a small voice in my head say, "Carolyn, this isn't going to go down well."

I returned to the surgicenter and with the NPP tucked under my arm, I stepped up to the front desk. "May I speak with your privacy official?"

The woman at the front desk said, "We don't have one."

"Of course you do," I responded. "It says so right here."

"Well, she's out on a coffee break."

"I can wait."

"Well, actually privacy is managed in our administrative offices." *Lies, lies.*

"Where are they located? I'm very concerned about my husband, and I need to file a complaint. I could file one with your privacy official or with the Secretary of HHS. Which is better for you?" I didn't raise my voice. I simply stated my rights as a family member and a caregiver. I also wanted to be sure my husband and I spoke with the doctor when he came out of the procedure.

"Just a moment," she said. "I'll let you speak with our nurse manager."

What I learned in the next few minutes amazed me.

The doctors didn't have time to wait for the family to be called back between each procedure, and that's why they asked the nurses to explain postsurgical procedures when the family member was present.

The nurses were so backed up that the only time they could talk to the family member was when they pulled around the back of the facility to pick up the patient.

Nurses identified themselves as the "patient advocate" while the patient was coming out of anesthesia, and the doctor took family members into a private room only when a biopsy indicated a positive malignancy.

"You have got a lot of things going on here," I said.

"You are right. This started out as a scheduling problem, and it just snowballed into a bigger quality concern for all the nurses. If you would file a complaint, I know we would be able to make some changes."

The nurse manager wrote down my comments, and I signed the document before my husband came out of anesthesia. My next biggest surprise was that before I left the facility, family members were invited to come back into the post-op room to speak with the physician about the procedure. Some were even invited into a private room to have a detailed conversation with the doctors.

(Carolyn Hartley)

HIPAA and Medical Identity Theft

In 2015, President Obama, the FBI, and the Department of Homeland Security identified medical identity theft as one of the top five critical components of the nation's infrastructure. Laws were in place to protect privacy, but breaches against Sony Pictures, Hollywood actors, Target, Home Depot, Anthem, Nordstrom, and others set the nation in a new direction for protecting an individual's identity. Medical identities are much more valuable on the black market than are credit cards. Health information will continue to become more personalized. Thieves can use your loved one's medical identity to obtain high-priced drugs for specialty treatment, purchase services from a hospital, and much more.

Watch for signs that you or your loved one are a victim of medical identity theft. These may include the following:

- An invoice from a hospital for services in another state or locally that you did not receive

- Incorrect listings of services on an explanation of benefits

- Invoices that arrive more than six months after the death of a loved one

- Denial of insurance coverage because of a medical condition you don't have

- Collection calls for medical services you did not receive

To launch an investigation, use your rights and ask for the following:

- A complete invoice that includes a breakdown of all billing codes. This may be a thirty-page document, but get it.

- An accounting of disclosures of all people who created, modified, or viewed your medical chart.

- Ask to speak to the organization's privacy official immediately. In a small practice, this also may be the practice administrator.

If you are not immediately satisfied with your investigation, you should take the following steps:

- With documentation in hand, file a complaint with the Federal Trade Commission at www.FTCcomplaintassistant.gov or call (877) ID-THEFT ([877] 438-4338).

- File a complaint with your state's attorney general. Do an Internet search for "state attorney general" and then your state to find the one in your state. All states have a portal for filing a complaint and a phone number to speak to a live person.

- Contact your local police.

- Call the OCR and file a complaint.

HIPAA and Personal Representatives

The rights of caregivers gained tremendous momentum in the early to mid-2000s when the nation faced damaging hurricanes and terrorist attacks. Immediately following 9/11, when terrorists attacked New York, Pennsylvania. and Washington, D.C., hospital administrators cited fear of HIPAA privacy penalties if they shared the whereabouts of victims who had been brought into the hospital. Families were frantic, trying to figure out where their loved ones had been transported. Public outcries immediately exploded about how much the federal government should intrude into citizens' lives to protect them and especially in a disaster.

In 2005, when Hurricanes Katrina and Rita wreaked havoc along the Gulf coast, hospital administrators and privacy officials again blocked the release of PHI, citing penalties and fear of privacy breaches. The Department of Health and Human

Services quickly released a Hurricane Katrina bulletin that put caregivers on the front lines. The bulletin notified health care providers to share patient information as necessary to locate and identify family members, guardians, or anyone else in the individual's care.

Building on lessons learned from these disasters, HHS and the OCR quickly published guides that permitted health care providers to communicate with family and friends, including personal representatives acting as caregivers. As caregivers, both authors downloaded this memo onto their smartphones in the event we needed to serve as refreshing educators.

Who Is Exempt from HIPAA?

Some organizations do not have to follow HIPAA laws. Law enforcement agencies do not need to seek written permission to access your medical records, but they are required to specify what they are seeking from your doctor or hospital. Your health care professional is required to document the request.

Examples of organizations that do not have to follow the HIPAA Privacy and Security Rules include the following:

- Life insurers

- Workers' compensation carriers

- Most schools and school districts

- Many state agencies, such as child protective service agencies

- Many municipal offices

To learn more about your privacy rights, use our Cool Tools.

Cool Tools

- Communication with Friends and Family: This tool comes straight from the OCR and provides guidance for when a health care practice, hospital, or dentist can share medical information with caregivers.

- Personal Representative: Most health care practices and hospitals will offer you their own form. An example from CIGNA is provided for you in Cool Tools.

- Health Care Durable Power of Attorney: If your loved one does not have a health care durable power of attorney, the state is likely to step in and force physicians to use extraordinary measures, even if your loved one wishes to be withdrawn from life support.

Additional Caregiver Rights: Family Medical Leave Act

Caregiving is an unpredictable profession. Often you are forced to make a moment-to-moment decision whether to leave work and take care of a family member or stay at work to keep your job. The Family Medical Leave Act, signed into law by President Clinton in 1993, requires employers with more than fifty employees to offer twelve weeks of medical leave during a twelve-month period to care for a son, daughter, or parent if that person has a serious health condition. Depending on the employer, you may not be paid during that twelve-week period, but you will have a position with the organization when you return. As baby boomers continue to age, the need for caregivers has created a need for stronger employment and public health policies.

If you are employed by an organization that has more than fifty employees or is otherwise large enough to hire or outsource a human resources department, you will likely find the most help from human resources and its employee policies and procedures. If you find you cannot get the help you need to obtain medical leave or fear that you will not be offered a position when you return, you may need the assistance of an attorney specializing in labor laws.

Additional Caregiver Rights:
Centers for Medicare and Medicaid Services (CMS)

If you are accessing Medicare or Medicaid funds to pay for your loved one's care at a nursing home (also called a skilled nursing facility), the Centers for Medicare and Medicaid Services (CMS) provides funds to state governments to oversee the licensing of nursing homes. States have an obligation to monitor nursing homes to ensure that they provide services in a safe, healthy, and clean environment. Depending on the problem, CMS can take action against the nursing home and stop providing funds if it loses its certification. If you believe that your loved one has been abused or that safety is in jeopardy, you have several rights you may use that we include in Cool Tools.

Cool Tools for Nursing Home Rights

- Nursing Home Compare: This is an invaluable tool to learn how your nursing home stacks up against other nursing homes. Reported deficiencies indicate areas where investigators requested or required a problem to be fixed to continue receiving funding.

- The Nursing Home Checklist: This is a great checklist when you are evaluating a nursing home.

- Administration on Aging: If you believe that a loved one is being abused at a long-term care facility, the best plan of action is to report the incident to the nursing home administrator and keep a record of that discussion. If you are not satisfied with the results, you may need to call 911 to report the abuse if you believe it is urgent. You may also consult with the National Center for Elder Abuse for help (part of the Administration on Aging).

Cool Tools That May Influence Your Rights at Work

The National Alliance for Caregiving is an organization that conducts in-depth studies on the impact of caregiving in the workplace. Organizations often use these studies to develop best practices in the workplace or influence labor laws for caregivers on the state and national levels. Our favorites include the following:

- Best Practices in Workplace Eldercare: Offer this document to your human resources department to help develop best practices for employed caregivers.

- The MetLife Study of Caregiving Costs to Working Caregivers—Double Jeopardy for Baby Boomers Caring for the Parents: Study defines the costs that working caregivers bear to support loved ones and benefits that employers can consider to enhance presenteeism to these caregivers.

- Caregivers of Veterans: As our veterans return home from war, many need continued care in the home or hospital. This somewhat dated study provides details on the types of injuries and the long-term care required from caregivers.

- CIGNA Personal Representative Form: This is an example of one insured's form. Be sure to get any form notarized or use one developed by your attorney.

Key Takeaways

In this chapter, you learned the following:

- You and your loved one have rights to privacy and confidentiality.

- Health care professionals can share information about your treatment with each other without your permission. They also can file a claim for reimbursement with your health plan unless you pay for the service out of pocket and ask to withhold information.

- If you think your rights or the confidential rights of your loved one have been violated, you can file a complaint with the practice, hospital, or the Secretary of HHS. The health care entity cannot retaliate against you.

- In an emergency, caregivers need to know their rights so that they can immediately connect with their loved one.

09 | Legal and Ethical Planning

Both legal and ethical planning are required for the protection of the caregiver and the loved one. Legal planning is needed to identify, sequence, and mitigate the risks to the caregiver as well as the patient. For this reason, you should consider consulting with an elder care attorney to be educated and advised of the legal aspects of caregiving.

Ethical planning refers to the moral aspects of human conduct, personal character, and integrity of choices. Ethical issues arise in caregiving, as the loved one often lacks the ability to make sound decisions surrounding his or her care. Some of the dilemmas are in relationship to responsibilities, personal rights and obligations, and perceived freedom.

This chapter is the mainstay for nearly all caregiving guidebooks, and we believe it should be part of our key messages to you as well. We will explore the following:

- Definitions of legal terms and the process one goes through in managing your loved one's legal affairs.

- The critical medical, legal, and financial documents needed to support your loved one.

- Ethical planning in caregiving.

Legal Planning for the Caregiver

Ellen Goodman of the Conversation Project, whose purpose is to help people talk about their wishes for end-of-life care, says, "Make end-of-life decisions early. Don't wait for a diagnosis or until someone is in the ER."

One of the first things caregivers and their loved ones need to do is talk about planning for the future. Your loved ones may have the capacity to make informed decisions about their health and finances now, but in the future they may not have this ability. This is a good time to consult an elder care attorney.

An elder care attorney is a skilled lawyer who specializes in legal services for the elderly. Their areas of proficiency include the following:

- Providing general estate planning

- Planning for the management of assets

- Assisting with medical directive documents to prepare for the possibility of your loved one's becoming incapacitated

- Wills and trusts

- Retirement and Social Security benefits

- Medicare and Medicaid planning

- Tax planning

An elder care attorney will be able to help caregivers and loved ones understand and interpret the varying laws of their state. For example, marriage status, relocation, or a death in the family could impact the preparation and maintenance of your legal documents.

When Dad's health took a turn for the worse at the same time that Mom was diagnosed with breast cancer, I consulted with my friend Sue, an elder care attorney in North Carolina. Because my parents lived in Pennsylvania, Sue recommended that I begin my search for an elder care attorney by either visiting the website of the National Academy of Elder Law Attorneys (NAELA), which provides a directory of elder care attorneys in the United States, or by searching online for a certified elder law attorney (CELA) in my parents' town. At this point in time this was all new to me, like finding a whole new line of resources I could access.

I located the names of three local CELAs and sent them to my sister. She researched their references on the Web as well as with her attorney friends who lived in the same town. After choosing one that she felt best met our needs, she phoned his office and explained to his assistant our parents' health situation and need for guidance. This was the easy part. The hard part was gathering the documents needed prior to our meeting with the attorney, such as our parents' identification, insurance policies, financial documents, real estate holdings, military benefits, and current will or trusts. It took my mom a couple of weeks to locate them, get copies to the attorney's office, and set the initial free consultation date.

When my sister, brother, and mom met with the attorney, he presented an assessment of my parents' situation, strategies of what he could provide, insight into Medicare and Medicaid, and a price breakdown for each of his services. We were able to solidify our parents' wishes in case of future incapacitation and also update their will and set up the power of attorney. We were pleased with the attorney's expertise and obvious experience with people like my parents and appreciated his help in guiding us on our caregiving journey.

Lessons we learned:

1. You should stress the need for an elder care attorney with your loved ones, but it is important that they don't feel it's being forced on them.
2. A third-party adviser can sometimes state things the caregiver cannot. For example, although I worked with a big-four accounting firm for many years, Mom would not heed my advice. But she listened to the attorney.
3. Consider bringing another person with you and your loved one to medical and legal meetings, as having an extra set of ears helps with accountability. If possible, it is also helpful to have someone help your loved one gather documents.
4. Do not always agree with the attorney. Question why a service is needed and the level of previous experience in similar situations. With my parents, the attorney was correct in advising my mom to consolidate her real estate assets, but the timing he suggested was unrealistic.
5. Ask for a free first consultation. A good CELA will meet with you first to assess your situation before providing any planning services.

(Peter Wong)

Cool Tools

- *Legal considerations when facing incapacity:* Key questions and a glossary of legal and financial terms
- *Elder care locator:* A free service of the U.S. Administration on Aging to help people locate services for seniors and caregivers in any part of the country

An elder care attorney can help you and your loved one prepare essential legal documents as you plan for the future. According to the National Institutes of

Health, an agency of the U.S. Department of Health and Human Services, these documents fall into two basic categories:

- Health care and medical documents
- Financial management and estate planning documents

Health Care and Medical Documents

1. *Durable power of attorney for health care:* A document giving legal authority to a designated person (i.e., caregiver) to make health care decisions on behalf of the loved one. It is also known as a health care proxy. This means that the designated person, or agent, may authorize or refuse medical treatment for the loved one. This power is activated by the loved one's physician but goes into effect only once the loved one is unable to make decisions for him- or herself.

2. *Living will:* An advance directive that describes and instructs how the loved one wants his or her end-of-life health care managed. This means that your loved ones decide in advance, while of sound mind and body, the kind of medical care they desire to receive or have withheld in the event they are unable to make their wishes known, such as the use of a ventilator, feeding tube, or dialysis.

3. *Do not resuscitate form (DNR):* An advance directive that is provided to health care professionals to authorize your loved one's wish of not being resuscitated if the heart stops or if your loved one stops breathing. The DNR is placed in one's medical health record or chart and is signed by a physician.

Cool Tools

- *Durable power of attorney for health care:* Samples of durable power of attorney for health care forms for each state, for informational purposes only. Always use a qualified legal adviser.

- *Living will:* Samples of living will forms for each state, for informational purposes only. Always use a qualified legal adviser.

- *DNR form:* Samples of DNR forms for each state, for informational purposes only. Always use a qualified legal adviser.

Financial Management and Estate Planning Documents

1. *Financial power of attorney:* A document giving a designated person or persons the authority to make legal and financial decisions on behalf of

the loved one. As the caregiver, it is important to know what authority you do and do not have with the power of attorney.

2. *Living trust:* A document giving a designated person, also known as a trustee, the authority to hold and distribute property and funds for the loved one once he or she is no longer capable of managing finances.

3. *Will:* A document indicating how the loved one's assets and estate will be distributed among beneficiaries after the loved one's death.

Cool Tools

- *Living Trust by Legal Zoom:* Samples of living trust forms for each state, for informational purposes only. Always use a qualified legal adviser. These are from Legal Zoom; all applicable terms and conditions apply. Requires Adobe Acrobat to view.

- *What's in a Will:* Lists the key components of a will, for informational purposes only. Always use a qualified legal adviser.

Ethical Planning for the Caregiver

There is no simple answer to ethical dilemmas presented to caregivers, as they do their best to care for loved ones. Getting your loved one to recognize the need for help and accept it is a difficult task. No one wants to be reminded of getting older and being unable to care for him- or herself.

In our family, it all began when Dad, who lived in Pennsylvania, suffered an aortic aneurysm at age sixty. He had just finished a round of golf with friends when he collapsed on the golf course. His friends were able to get him into a car and rush him to the hospital. At home in Alabama, I received a phone call from my brother saying my family and I needed to come immediately and "bring funeral clothes." We were able to get a flight that day and arrived at the hospital after midnight. Dad was still in the emergency room. He was later moved to the critical care unit, where he remained for twenty-one days. I remember my sister-in-law's father, the hospital chief of staff, telling my family that he did not believe Dad would live.

Dad's health emergency had brought our family together, and we began trying to plan for the future. We faced a lot of uncomfortable issues and had many questions:

"What if Dad doesn't come out of the coma?"

"If Dad dies, what would his funeral wishes be?"

"If Dad lives, will he be incapacitated?"

"Will Dad need special care?"

- "Do we need to look into a different living arrangement for him, such as assisted living or a nursing home? You know he would never want to be in a nursing home."

- "How do we make that medical decision, and who makes the decision?"

- "Is it wrong to think that Dad may die? Does it mean my faith isn't very strong?"

- "Are my thoughts normal?"

- "How much is all this going to cost, and can we afford it?"

- "Does Dad have a will?"

- "What have other people done in this situation?"

Dad eventually recovered and was released from the hospital. He told us later that he had a near-death experience while being transported to the hospital in the backseat of his friend's car.

He vividly described "seeing a bright light and hearing a voice say it was not yet time for him to leave."

The voice continued, "I haven't seen you in church on Sundays."

Dad told us that he replied, "I've been on the golf course every week, but if I make it through this, I promise I will be in church every Sunday!"

This was a life-changing promise that Dad was happy to keep, and after his recovery, he faithfully accompanied my mom to church every Sunday morning and played golf in the afternoon.

Dad's health emergency was a wake-up call to our family. My family members are highly intelligent, strong leaders in their communities and the business world, but it didn't matter. We were all caught off guard. Going through this medical challenge with Dad showed us the importance of having critical legal documents completed and available so that, if necessary, we could know end-of-life wishes and follow them. We learned that when people are confronted with serious illness or death, there are many anxieties and stresses about tomorrow and how important it is to work together to help parents as they age.

In addition to the aortic aneurism, over the next twenty years, Dad endured severe pancreatitis, open-heart surgery, hyperkalemia (too much potassium in the blood), congestive heart failure, a stroke, pulmonary edema, partial blindness, diabetes, and arthritis. The family joke was that the hospital was planning to name a wing after Dad since he was such a frequent visitor. My mom was Dad's main caregiver through it all, honoring her marriage vow of "in sickness and in health, for better or for worse."

The tables were turned when Mom was diagnosed with breast cancer and had to have chemotherapy and radiation treatments. Dad became her caregiver and helped her through her recovery despite his own poor health. This was when my brother, sisters, and I located an elder care attorney and began the process of having legal documents for financial and health care power of attorney prepared for our parents. Mom and Dad already had a will and a living will, but we realized it was important for them to have additional help in making their everyday lives as stress free as possible.

The last few years really showed us the importance of planning ahead while both Mom and Dad were still capable of being a part of the decision-making process. The ethical issue for us was knowing the right time to step in and help them.

Our family went through the same difficult situations many of our readers have also experienced with loved ones. For me, it was the guilt I felt when I helped move Dad from the hospital to the rehab/nursing home as a part of his last recovery, knowing that he might not leave there and that he never wanted to be in a nursing home environment. Mom wanted him to go home, and Dad always thought he would go home, but he passed away at age eighty-one while in the rehab center.

(Peter Wong)

Common Ethical Issues of Caregivers

As a caregiver, you are faced with situations that may go against what another person or persons or the establishment believes. This is called an ethical dilemma and requires you to choose between two courses of action, neither of which seems totally right to all parties. Some of the ethical issues that may arise can include the following:

- *When to prolong life:* People are living longer than ever before due to the availability of new medicines and technologies. Sometimes this puts a caregiver in the dilemma of choosing to prolong the loved one's life at the expense of his or her quality of life. An interesting study of physicians asked if they would want a DNR order in place if they had a terminal illness. The majority answered yes, they would not want to be resuscitated, since they understood firsthand that prolonging one's life had no bearing on one's quality of life.

- *The sanctity of life:* This is the belief that human life has value at every age. For example, if your loved one has no hope for health improvement and feels there is no longer a reason to live, he or she may consider taking his or her own life. The ethical issue arises if a physician is asked to assist the suicide, which goes against the medical principle of "do no harm."

- *Durable power of attorney:* This gives legal authority to make medical decisions on behalf of the loved one. Many times it is the caregiver who is given this authority. An ethical dilemma can arise when a decision made for your loved one differs from what family members want for whatever reasons (guilt or religious beliefs). There are no easy answers to these situations.

- *Nursing home versus at-home care:* What do you do if your loved ones are unable to care for themselves? What if your love one needs a higher level of care than you can provide at home? How do you balance the acceptance of your loved one's vehement distaste of nursing homes with the knowledge that it seems to be the best answer for quality care? You may feel guilt regardless of your choice of action. "I Promised My Parents I'd Never Put Them in a Nursing Home" is a blog that discusses this issue.

- The key in all of this is good communication within your family. "Being able to politely and effectively discuss difficult issues can keep relationships with relatives strong," says Agingcare.com, "in spite of the challenges that arise when caring for an aging adult." Some of the topics you will want to discuss include the following:

The current status of your loved one's health/medical report. Consult chapter 8 if you have difficulty accessing your loved one's medical report.

Who can be the primary caregiver for your loved one?

Will your loved one be able to continue living at home, or will you need to review other living arrangements?

What are the estimated costs of your loved one's care (what does insurance cover, and who pays any remaining costs)? How will you divide costs after your loved one passes away? Consult chapter 7 to learn more about managing medical bills.

Will family members need to share the financial responsibility of your loved one's care?

Cool Tools

- *Family Caregiver Alliance:* One of the best websites for research, information, advocacy, and support of caregivers.

- *National Institute on Aging Information Center:* Publishes the following:

  - *Agepage: Getting Your Affairs in Order*

  - *Advance Care Planning: Tips from the National Institute on Aging*

  - *End of Life: Helping with Comfort and Care*

  - *So Far Away: Twenty Questions and Answers about Long-Distance Caregiving*

- *Alzheimer's Disease Education and Referral Center (ADEAR):* Provides information for families, caregivers, and health care professionals on care treatments, education and training, and research on Alzheimer's disease. Many of the caregiver's processes and information are transferable to other caregiving illnesses. Discusses relevant legal and ethical issues regarding long-term illnesses of your loved ones.

Completing Your Ethical Planning: Frequently Asked Questions

Who should lead your ethical planning process? If your loved one is mentally capable, he or she can guide the process. Otherwise, it should be one who is trusted by the loved one. Many times this will be the caregiver since he or she is usually closest to the loved one and best understands the daily physical, mental, and spiritual needs to communicate to your attorney and family members. Sometimes an objective person, such as a close family friend or minister or rabbi, may be the best person. The loved one, caregiver, and family members should all be invited to the ethical planning discussions with your elder care attorney, but not everyone will want to be involved, and some may not choose to attend. It is important to respect one's decision to be excluded and not hold it against him or her in the future.

Are ethical plans legal documents? Not always. But there are essential legal documents within an ethical plan that your elder care attorney will assist you with, such as advance directives, durable power of attorney for health care, DNR, and medical proxy. If you do not document your loved one's wishes legally, there is no guarantee that the wishes will be carried out. Allow your loved one's legal documents to dictate the course of action.

What if family members disagree? Family members will disagree at some point during the ethical planning process, whether because of religious beliefs or just having different thoughts about the loved one's wishes. Let everyone's voice be heard, but remember that it is important for you, the caregiver, to have thick skin and not take things personally. You cannot make everyone happy, especially in difficult decision-making situations. Once your loved one's decisions have been expressed and legally documented, your role is to execute the wishes with compassion.

How do you keep your loved one from feeling left out? Sometimes this happens unintentionally. Allow your elderly loved one to make his or her own decisions as much as possible and respect what is said.

What if you suspect that your loved one is not safe in the home? An ethical dilemma can arise if you are not able to make the home a safe living environment and must make a decision for other living arrangements against the will of your loved one.

> Dad had fallen and been taken to the emergency room for the third time in two months. It was becoming an obviously dangerous situation for both Mom and Dad. Remaining in the home was important for both of them, though, so after one of Dad's hospital and subsequent rehabilitation stays, we had the rehabilitation supervisor do a home safety assessment. This showed the family the constructive safety changes we needed to make in the house, such as removing their dog (a high fall risk) and rearranging furniture that obstructed foot traffic.
> (Peter Wong)

What if your loved one wants treatment that others in the family believe to be unethical (e.g., stem cell implants)? As the caregiver, it is your decision how to respond to the opinions of others. You may choose to ignore them, or you may want to thank them for their concerns. Ultimately, your responsibility is to follow the wishes of your loved one as much as possible.

Cool Tools

- *AgingCare.com:* A well-respected resource that discusses family caregiving and ethical situations. It is a meeting place that connects families, caregivers, and elder care experts.

- *Community Care:* An online resource in dealing with end-of-life planning and issues.

Key Takeaways

In this chapter, you learned the following:

- Legal and ethical planning protects both the caregiver and your loved one.

- You may want to work with an elder care attorney.

- Good communication between the caregiver, loved one, and family members is critical in resolving ethical dilemmas.

10 Putting Your Communication Plan to Work for You

Initially, most caregivers just want to get the word out about their loved one's status: "He's out of intensive care and been assigned a room. Not sure when he'll be home" or "She's stable. The doctors say she has a strong pulse. The family is coming home, and we need your help." A communication plan is your tool for keeping friends and family informed of your loved one's condition. As soon as you begin sharing details about your loved one's care with others, you have launched a communication plan. That is the way it should be. You and your hero need hugs, meals, prayers, and a helping hand. But after the first two or three weeks, friends are likely to stay out of your way, leaving the doors open to "call when you need help." This is when your communication plan benefits from a strategy. To start, make some initial decisions:

- Who needs to be made aware of your situation?
- Will you communicate via a Web portal, social networking site, e-mail, phone calls, or a combination of these?
- How often will you share information?
- How do you want friends to reach out to you?
- How much information do they want, and what do you want to give?
- How will you ask for help?

Let's start with background information and then move into a decision tool to build your plan.

Who Needs to Know?

One of the first things to decide is who needs to be informed of your situation and how you will communicate this information. Family and close friends are a no-brainer. For other friends and contacts, a "keep me updated" list often begins with a Christmas card list or personal telephone list in electronic form (smartphone) or paper address book, but even those lists need scrutiny. Some messages are much more emotional and meant to be shared with family, clergy, or close friends. Other messages are updates, such as "Mom had a great day today. We went out for lunch and sat in the park for more than an hour watching the grandkids play soccer." You may find that a communications form like the one in table 10.1 will help you keep family and friends informed of your loved one's situation.

What Format Will You Use to Communicate?

Social media makes for quick messaging and allows people to post updates online. Five years ago, most of us would not have considered Facebook, Twitter, LinkedIn, Pinterest, Google Plus, Instagram, or Bitly to be common forms of written communication. If you don't have a clue what this means, you aren't alone, but to manage

Table 10.1.   List of Key Contacts

Immediate Family Contact Information			
Who	**Phone**	**E-Mail**	**Address**
Mother			
Father			
Brother			
Sister			
Grandkids			
Extended Family			
Aunt			
Uncle			
Cousins			
Niece			
Nephew			
Friends from Work			
Church/Temple or Synagogue Friends			

communications using the Web, consider coordinating key messages with a family member who understands how to use these tools but also agrees to withhold sensitive information. Unless you have built security in to these sites (see chapter 3), these are publicly accessible ways to communicate. You may want friends to share your posts with other friends and family members, the real intent of social media, but once a message is posted, it takes on a life of its own. Our mothers would have called "posts" postcards where anyone can read what you wrote. This may be considered an invasion of privacy by some, while others call it "sharing." Consult your loved one's wishes before posting public information.

Another way to communicate is through a secure messaging portal where you control who has access and what they can do with the information you post. We discuss these portals in this chapter, but a short list includes the following:

Caringbridge.org
Dailystrength.org
Carepages.org

Websites like these are usually free but are supported by donations or ads.

One of my first AMA coauthors moved his family to Minnesota to join a major firm as its chief privacy officer. Mike worked diligently to legally protect his clients and was highly favored among government, medical, and legal communities. His friends, family, church, and business colleagues celebrated his achievements because he also gave back more than he received.

Six months after he moved, my friend was diagnosed with pancreatic cancer. Mike had everything going for him—a national reputation and relationships with federal appointees—but most important to him were his beautiful wife and children. He poured such love into his family that it was nearly impossible to think of a disease manifesting itself in such a remarkably humble but successful man.

Mike, his wife, and children, now 1,000 miles away, agreed to share some of their joy, treatment updates, and frustrations as they journeyed through his cancer treatment. They built a site on a secure website, Caringbridge.org, to allow family and friends access to their Web postings.

While the family diligently guarded his privacy, visitors to the site could scroll through weeks of letters, blogs, and quips of praise written by friends and family. It was easy to add a sentence or two to cajole and uplift his spirits.

Sometimes the daily blog was brief: "Tough day."

On other days, the blog entry was enough to let us know our friend was resting and watching old movies.

Something happened along the way to my website posts. I began to feel like I was part of the caring team. While I never spent a moment inside the home, I also knew that his family graciously shared some intimate, caring moments with us. I was sitting in the room with the family without physically imposing myself or interrupting precious conversations.

A few days before Mike turned fifty, his wife and children launched a massive website campaign asking readers to send humorous birthday cards. With joy, Mike's wife "complained" in her blog about having to carry more than 500 cards to his bedside.

A few short weeks later, she and her children wrote a tribute to him that we wouldn't be privileged to know if Mike's wife and family hadn't carefully shared portions of their lives with us.

(Carolyn Hartley)

If time is of the essence for you, getting the message out will be easier with a secure portal. Other formats include e-mail, telephone, and old-fashioned letters.

If you choose to use social media, send invitations to many people to join your invitation-only network. There are several great tools for learning how to communicate using social media. Our favorites include The Internet for the Older and Wiser: Get Up and Running Safely on the Web and The Moz Blog: The Free Beginners Guide to Social Media.

Cool Tools for Long-Distance Caregivers

If you have been legally named your loved one's personal representative in a durable power of attorney or health care power of attorney, your communication processes will be a little more challenging between home visits. Both authors put plenty of miles on our frequent-flyer programs taking care of parents who lived far away. We know your challenges. You can still pull together a communication plan, but need to be a little more creative.

One Web-based communications tool, Voice-Over-Internet Protocol (VOIP), allows you to see the person while talking to them. A few are listed for you here:

■ *Skype:* Skype is one of the most well-known tools, and approximately 600 million people have used the program. As with most VOIP software, you will need a computer with a webcam (Web-based camera) that is built in to the computer.[1] Avoid putting any confidential information over Skype. As it is widely used, it is not secure.

- *FaceTime:* FaceTime is an application originally built for Apple computer products, such as iPhones, Macintosh computers, and iPads. FaceTime is a free app that allows users on both end to visually and audibly communicate with each other. Similar applications are available for Android and Microsoft smartphones.

- *Toll-free numbers:* Nearly all mobile or landline telephone providers offer 800-type capabilities, and some offer them for free, but you pay the cost from each person who uses your toll-free number. A nonprofit organization, Tollfreenumber.org, can help if your phone company's fees are too high.

My parents lived in a small rural town in northern Missouri, close enough to civilization to purchase groceries and building supplies but not at all connected to broadband or wireless Internet capabilities. When I remarried and moved away, most of their friends commented that I had abandoned my eighty-year-old parents at a time when they needed me most. Hard as I tried to get them to move with me, my parents were settled and wouldn't budge. On my next trip home, before the abandonment conversation started up again, I provided my new 800 telephone number to their friends and asked them to "please call me on this line in the event you think my parents need help." Only one or two of them had cell phones, and most were reluctant to pay the cost of a long-distance call from a landline. We bonded instantly—not only that I had provided a number but also that I brought them into my caregiving communication plan. None ever abused the 800 line, but when they thought my parents needed help, I got a call. I always told the friend how grateful I was that they took the time to alert me to a potential health issue.
    (Carolyn Hartley)

How Often Will You Share Information?

Start by taking a look at your calendar to evaluate how much time you can spend communicating with friends and family. In the absence of communication, people

---

1. The authors do not recommend using VOIP software with an older computer that does not have a built-in webcam, as the download and installation process frequently causes the computer's operating system to lock up.

often miscommunicate, resulting in rumors or hurt feelings that take more time to correct, manage, and heal.

Initially, let's say you will post your message once a week on Sunday evenings. Of course, you may choose any time or day of the week, but the point is that you set a regular time to update your messages.

How Do You Want Friends to Reach Out to You?

Your communication plan should not be so rigid that it prevents people you want to see from coming to you. You know your friends, and you know how they like to share with you:

- *In person:* Some may want to bring a meal and offer comforting words to you. Let them.

- *Phone call:* Others may call you and ask how you are doing. Bring it on. If this isn't a good time for a call, learn how to use a Cool Tool on your smartphone that allows you to create instant-response messages to the caller. These messages can be customized, but standard messages generally include the following:

  "I can't take your call but will call you back shortly."
  "Currently on another call. May I call you back?"
  "Thanks for your call. I'll get back to you in a bit."

Social Media and Secure Portals

You may feel you are putting distance between you and your friends if you ask them to post a message on a social media site. Get started by "priming the pump." Ask one or two friends to post a message, then respond to the sender or click "Like" on the message. This serves as an encouraging example to others that they also can communicate with you and that you are reading the message.

Portals are excellent for friends who also tend to whine about themselves when you call for help. You know who they are. As if you had time to comfort them, suddenly you are listening to their pains, their children's problems, or their spousal relationships. This isn't a one-time event, but every time you are in a conversation with them, you will be on the phone for an hour listening to the same old stories. There will be a time and a place to exchange supportive chatter, but secure communication portals are terrific for these friends who you don't want to lose but who you just don't have the energy at the moment to help.

Manage the Information You Will Provide and What You Won't Provide

In chapter 3, we provided guidance on how to build your personal and family records. Medical, social, and family history details that you included in personal health record tools are confidential and should *not* be shared in a public forum. Let's take a look at what you do and do not want to provide through social media. *Do* provide the following:

- How you are doing, for example a few words from your journals, how you feel, or reminders about how grateful you are to friends and family.

- For children with special needs, provide guidance on toys to bring and games your child enjoys.

- How your loved one is doing; for example, "Mom is resting well today, but last night was really tough for her." Additional messages are provided at the end of this chapter.

- Where to send messages.

- What times your loved one is available to meet with friends.

- General requests for help, but direct respondents to an e-mail, not a phone number.

- Names of charities for donations.

- Names of local florists.

- Names of local restaurants that provide carryout.

- Links to Cool Tools at the end of this chapter.

Do *not* provide the following:

- Any personal information, such as street addresses, phone number, or birth date.

- Banking information. If you are setting up a foundation, consult an attorney to set up the foundation. Also consult a certified public accountant to coordinate how funds will be managed and disbursed with your bank.

- Medications. If you need someone to pick up a prescription medication for you, call that person or send a text. In most states, the pharmacy will require in writing the name of individuals outside the family you have assigned permission to pick up medications.

How to Communicate When You Need Help

Caregivers tend to be either the best or the worst at asking for help. Don't over-think the request. You aren't admitting that you are weak when asking for help. No need to apologize. Your house doesn't need to be in order for someone to stop by and help. Best of all, you are giving someone who really wants to be involved in your life an opportunity to help. Let them in.

Toni Bernhard, J.D., writes in *Psychology Today* to turn the request for help into an experiment. She admits that she often forgot to follow up on her previous offers to help others. But when she became chronically ill, she interpreted other people's offers to help as insincere. In her lessons learned, Bernhard says it's just the opposite:

1. When people offer to help, they mean it. Friends don't like to be helpless.
2. The responsibility to follow up falls on the caregiver or loved one.
3. Give them a specific task to do, for example, "Can you help with my laundry every other week?"

We've worked through details of your strategic communication plan. Now let's go to table 10.2 and put the plan into a tool that works for you.

When Communication Needs Quick Response

Your communications planning becomes your vital tool when you need it most. In the event of an emergency, use the following outline to help convey key messages to your family:

A. The current situation
   Here is what happened.
B. If help is needed, what action should be taken?
   Physical help
      Meals
      Cleaning
      Errands
      Driving to appointments
   Emotional help
      Visitation
   Spiritual help
      Prayer
C. What is the best way to communicate back to the family?

Table 10.2. Build Your Communication Plan

Communication	Who Takes the Lead	With Help from
Social media:		
Secure Web portals		
Facebook, Twitter, etc.?		
Letters		
Phone	(See table 10.1 for a list of key contacts.)	
Frequency		
How often will we post?		
Types of messages:		
Caregiver journals		
Loved one's journals		
Ask for help		
How Family Can Be Reached		
Caregiver	E-mail? Phone? When not to call	
Caregiver's delegated representative		
Emergency Information/Rapid Deployment		
Key contact	Tool to access (table 10.4)	

E-mail

Phone/text

Phone/voice mail

Our family posted the following announcement on Caringbridge.org for friends and family who had been following Dad's care:

Hello Wong Family:

I wanted to update you on the current situation with Dad. He suffered an aortic aneurism last night. He is stable and is in the intensive care unit at York Hospital in York, Pennsylvania. Dad will be in intensive care until further notice, with the next 48 hours being the most critical. A lot of waiting and praying.

All the children are coming in and staying at either the house or the Courtyard Marriott on Queen Street. Mom is staying with Dad at the hospital. We can be reached via cell phone at xxx-xxx-xxxx. Leonard will be on point for any questions during this time.

Key updates on Dad will be posted on CaringBridge.org.

Thank you for your prayers,

Debbie, Leonard, Susan, and Peter

In this case, the Wong family needed to quickly disburse multiple roles. Table 10.3 shows how those roles were assigned and tracked.

Looking back at our family's health situation with Dad, our family followed this chart 80 percent of the time for communicating updates via the Caringbridge. org blog site. The other 20 percent of our time was spent phoning rather than e-mailing. While e-mails and updating Dad's blog were efficient for getting out the message, we found it healing to speak with our relatives and close friends personally by phone, as they wanted to hear from us firsthand and express their love and concern. Using Caringbridge.org as a means to update the masses of friends was very efficient, and it was also comforting for Mom to read the response messages that many friends posted there.

(Peter Wong)

Table 10.4 provides a blank tool you can use to build your own rapid-deployment plan, especially when the situation requires delegation to trusted friends and family. Use content in table 10.3 to guide you with ideas.

Cool Tools That Keep You Updated

- Caringbridge.org is a nonprofit organization that connects friends, family, and loved ones in a secure Web-hosted environment. To get started, you create a free site and establish privacy privileges, enabling guests to see

Table 10.3. Completed Sample Communication Plan

Distribution Person	Topic/Message	Communication Vehicle	Frequency	Audience	Completed
Brother	Update on Dad	CaringBridge.org	Daily/as needed	Family/friends/coworkers	Yes
Self	Meals for Mom	TakeThemAMeal.com	Once a week	Church	Yes
Brother	Patient data; drug update	E-mail	As needed	Family physician, cardiologist	Yes
Brother	Rental properties	E-mail/phone	Once a week or as needed	Immediate family	Yes
Brother	Hospice preparations	E-mail/phone	Once a week on Monday afternoon	Physician and hospice	Yes
Self	Insurance and medical billing	E-mail/phone	Bimonthly	Self and brother	Ongoing
Sister	Power of attorney	E-mail/phone	Monthly	Brother and sister	Ongoing

Table 10.4.   Rapid-Deployment Plan

Distribution Person	Topic/Message	Communication Vehicle	Frequency	Audience	Completed

all posts and also post comments, or you can restrict access by requiring visitors to sign up on log-on to your site. For greater privacy, you can allow only guests you invite onto the site to view your entries. Most people select medium level of privacy. You also can allow people to search for the site by entering the individual's name on the Caringbridge site.

- Posthope.org and Carepages.com are sites similar to Caringbridge. We like Caringbridge because it is funded by donations and does not allow advertising, and the system designers block search engines from accessing and sharing details, such as private posts and user IDs.

Communication Examples

Share with your health care provider any medical event you have experienced outside their network. Remember to update any other health care professional, such as your pharmacist and dentist. Examples of a letter/fax used to communicate to a physician regarding updating a patient's health care file and adverse reaction to medication are provided in the following pages. You can send similar information through your patient portal as described in chapter 3.

Communication with Your Health Care Professional

Communicating with your health care professional and understanding what your clinician has said is imperative to the long-term care of your loved one. There may be instances when a patient or caregiver meets with a health care professional and the following happens:

1. The patient or caregiver may not understand the diagnosis and is afraid to ask.
2. The patient or caregiver may not understand the care instructions being given due to feeling overwhelmed by the situation.
3. The patient or caregiver only partially remembers the care instructions.
4. The patient hears only what he or she wants to hear.
5. The patient or caregiver, whether purposefully or not, does not communicate the correct message for care to other family members.

Why not carry a tape recorder to capture the conversation? Many smart devices have built-in applications or recording capabilities. Some digital recorders and smart devices also have the ability to store discussions on your personal computer for reference or to share with family members via e-mail. We have found that a recording device is a practical way to document discussions and understand the next steps for the patient.

Figure 10.1.   Letter to Update Patient's Health Care File

Dr. XXXX
Northeast Medical Center, Ste 2000
Concord, NC 28026

Dear Dr. XXXX:

Please ensure that updated information is placed in the patient health care file of xxxxx xxxxx. I have included a copy of the information from his/her emergency room visit while in Colorado in June 2014. His/her physician was Dr. Peter Wong, Internal Medicine, 10200 Trail West Blvd., Buena Vista, Colorado 28003.

I am the caregiver for this individual and on the HIPAA list for him/her.

Kind Regards,

xxxxxxx

Figure 10.2. Sample Message to Update the Patient's Adverse Reaction to Medication

Paula Smith, Pharmacist
CVS Pharmacy
24000 Popular Tent Rd.
Concord, NC 28207

Dear Paula:

Please update Peter Wong's drug history file. His birth date is xx-xx-xxxx.

He was recently given penicillin 300 mg and had a severe reaction.

Kind Regards,

Peter Wong
HIPAA on file

We recommend that you explain to the health care professional why you would like to record the discussion. It is a means of correctly capturing the information and is not for liability reasons. Be aware that recording another person without permission may be illegal in your state.

We also suggest that the caregiver have another family member or close friend accompany him or her on follow-up visits with the health care professional to help the caregiver remember what has been said.

Cool Tools for Communication

- *Caringbridge.org:* A Web-based tool to help connect family and friends during a health event.

- *Carepages.com:* A Web-based tool to help connect family and friends during a health event.

- *Myfamily.com:* A Web-based tool; a small fee applies for blog usage.

- *Dailystrength.org:* A share forum in a secure communication process among friends and family.

- *TakeThemAMeal.com:* A Web-based tool to simplify meal coordination so that friends, family, neighbors, and coworkers can show that they care.

- *Patientslikeme.com:* A Web-based tool to share your experience, give and get support, and improve your life and the lives of others. Compare treatments, symptoms, and experiences with people like you.

- *HealthinAging.org:* A resource article on improving communication with your provider from the Health in Aging Foundation.

- *Kinnexxus.com:* A Web-based fee service used for communication, connecting adults, friends, family, and professional care providers with the caregiver.

Key Takeaways

In this chapter, you learned the following:

- When building your communication plan, make a list of who needs to know what and when they need to know it.

- Communicate via secure Web portal, social networking site, e-mail, or phone calls, always respecting your loved one's privacy.

- Decide how often you will share information.

- Decide who will field questions from friends and distant relatives.

- Build a list of tasks that need to be completed; leave it in an open place for people to volunteer.

Risk Management and Documentation Plan

Now that you've gathered Cool Tools and can securely access information to make your caregiving life more rewarding, you need a plan in the event an electronic device is lost or stolen. It's called a risk management plan. A risk management plan begins by asking a lot of "what if" questions. What if no one knows how to log in to Mom's online bank account? What if your husband loses his smartphone that contains unsecure medical information? What if someone steals your phone or handheld device, such as an iPad? In all these cases, your identity has been stolen, creating havoc for you while you are caring for your loved one. The management portion, then, is to develop a plan that eliminates the problem or that helps minimize the impact on you.

In this chapter, we will review two areas of backup planning, or risk management:

- How to plan for the loss of key data, for example, on your mobile device. Both the caregiver and the loved one need each other to have a plan in place.

- How to make a backup documentation plan.

What If My Smartphone Is Lost or Stolen?

As the caregiver, you may have all your loved one's important contacts on your smartphone. For example, you may keep photos of the insurance card, Veterans Administration card, and Medicare card on your phone or handheld device. You may also have contact numbers and addresses of your loved one's physicians, home health care, and rehab centers in addition to all of the important medical appointment dates you are helping to keep track of. Then one day as you are winding down your day's activities, you plug in the charger but cannot find the smartphone. You empty pockets, shake purses, and recount where you've been in the past five hours. You call your mobile phone but cannot hear the ring. Sleep? Not happening.

Has it been lost? Stolen? Your digital secretary is no longer with you, and you have no clue about tomorrow's schedule let alone how to shut down the phone.

According to myPhoneMD, there are five important actions to take if your phone is lost or stolen:

1. Notify your mobile provider to disable your phone as soon as possible to prevent any unwanted long-distance charges or unwanted e-mails sent to your contacts:

   Sprint lost/stolen phone information
   Verizon lost/stolen phone information
   AT&T lost/stolen phone information

   You will need the phone number and password for the account. You may be required to send a copy of the power of attorney to the carrier if the phone belonged to your loved one.

2. Change all online passwords for any accounts linked to the device (e.g., e-mail accounts, personal health records, bank accounts, bill payments, and so on).

3. Go online and activate your device's tracking software. This was initially used to track and monitor younger family members, but many caregivers are now placing this on their loved one's smartphone. Tracking software is also commonly used by law enforcement to find those who have stolen your smartphone.

4. Alert family and friends that your or your loved one's smartphone was stolen. (They may get a phone call or e-mail from the phone and need to know it is not coming from you.)

5. Contact the carrier insurance if you have purchased insurance on the device.

Cool Tools

- *AT&TFamilyMaps:* Device tracker for AT&T devices. First thirty days are free.

- *FindMyiphone:* Device tracker for iPhones, iPads, iPods, or Mac. Free.

- *MyPlanB:* Android tool that will assist you if you did not have tracking device software on your phone. Free.

- *Lookout:* Android and iPhone device tracking and other security features. $3 per month.

My mom, who was notorious in our family for losing items, recently took an Amtrak train to visit my sister four hours away. After she arrived there, I received a text from my sister saying that Mom could not find her wallet. Did Mom leave it on the Amtrak? Did someone steal it? We have prayed many times, "Lord, give us patience and help us find Mom's (missing item of the moment)." In this particular instance, there was a happy ending when Mom later "found" the wallet exactly where she had placed it. The problem was that she didn't remember putting it inside her carry-on bag because she always puts it in an outside pocket of her bag.

This time it was Mom's wallet, but it could've easily been her phone as it has been in the past. Thankfully it had not been stolen, and fortunately we have a backup plan with copies of all her important information from both her wallet and her phone.

As a caregiver, you could easily substitute the name of your loved one into this story because it is something you most likely have dealt with also.

(Peter Wong)

I (Peter) have personal experience not only within my family with risk management but also in my professional background working with the Federal Bureau of Investigation and the Cyber Task Force for the Secret Service. People may think they are aware of what happens when a phone is lost or stolen, but many times the true consequences are not seen until much later.

For example, in meetings with federal and state law enforcement officials, our discussions have centered on the high number of universities whose students have been victims of a common cybercrime: identity theft. The customary response to identity theft is to sign up for credit reports and check them a couple of times a year to see if any fraudulent activity has occurred. When no activity is seen over a couple of years, the victim believes his or her identity is safe. For example, criminals may initially choose college students as their first targets. Then the students graduate, and, say, ten years later, many are in the prime of their income brackets and business professions. It is at this point when the criminals will use the stolen identities and wreak havoc on the unsuspecting victims.

Another identity theft target preyed on is the elderly. Criminals recognize that older people do not have the best security habits, nor do they keep track of items as well as they once did. They may have larger assets and do not always have a detailed backup plan in place.

In New York City alone, a phone is lost or stolen every three seconds. So the best security method is to put a plan in place and make it part of your everyday life. As the caregiver for your loved one, make it a habit to check his or her credit reports a couple of times each year. Also make certain that you have backed up the important information located on your loved one's smartphone. Have a practice drill with your caregiver or loved one and follow our suggestions to ensure that both of you know what to do.

We hope that you or your loved one will never be in this situation, but it is still wise to practice good risk management. What does that mean?

As I instructed my teenage children many years ago, it means you think about a situation in advance and plan ahead in the event the situation does happen. As my Boy Scout leader would say, "Be prepared. That means you!"

Plan now with your smartphone or device:

- *Secure your data:* Put a password on your device and make sure the code is not the typical 1234 or 0000. Do not use an anniversary date or a birthday. Ensure that it is easy for your loved one to remember but difficult for others to duplicate. For example, use phrases along with numbers: Psalms 23 = GreenPastures23. Or relate passwords to sports, such as I love to play golf = ILuv2playgolf.

- *Ensure that your e-mail and social media accounts (e.g., Facebook and Twitter) have passwords:* Always log out of your accounts so that no one can replicate your identity and post vulgar or nondiscreet pictures, among other things, from your smartphone. For example, you may have read in the media about someone finding or stealing a smartphone and sending e-mails to the victim's entire contact list asking for money. The readers of the e-mails recognize the sender's name, open the e-mail, and become victims of fraud if they respond to it. An example of using social media accounts on your smartphone is a picture or comment sent out on Twitter or Facebook that is not from you.

- *Back up your information:* Photos, contact lists, and current apps are gone forever if you lose your smartphone and it is not backed up. The typical backup procedure for iPhone and Android is easy. Just plug your smartphone into your computer with your USB cord. You can also use services like iCloud for the iPhone or GCloud for the Android. It is important that both the caregiver and the loved one back up the information stored on their smartphones.

- *Put the carrier's phone number in a safe place:* In the event your phone is lost or stolen, you will need your carrier's contact number to cancel your service. It may be good to place it in the glove compartment of your vehicle as a backup plan since many times the purse is stolen with the smartphone in the purse.

Finally, if you cannot locate your smartphone and you have a data backup plan already in place, you may want to wipe out all of your personal information. Many tracking device companies offer this service. Do this only if you are certain the device has been stolen and you have a data backup plan in place. The intent is to prevent others from gathering your personal information.

Making Your Backup Documentation Plan

An elder care attorney said that the most daunting experience after her husband's stroke was to reconstruct all the things that needed to be done and having to figure them out by herself. Dave, a former executive with UnitedHealth, said that after both he and his wife had life-threatening surgery, he pulled all his legal, financial, home security, and funeral wishes together into a Dropbox account, then gave each of his kids the complex user ID and password combination. "This is my 'I love you! box,'" Dave said. "I want to play golf for the rest of my life without worrying whether my kids can carry on without me."

Taking care of parents and advising friends in emergency situations with their loved ones has emphasized to us the importance of knowing the location of original documents and having copies of official records. Many do not know where to find their loved ones' original documents and aren't sure where to begin looking. With documentation, consider your risks by asking the following questions:

Identify the risks: What type of risk does it represent if I do not have the documents? How do I find the documents?

Determine the impact: What is the impact of not having the documents?

- *Financial risks:* Late-payment charges; incorrect billing; not having the military records could delay benefits for your loved one after death.

- *Health risks:* Possible inability to get proper care; medicine mix-ups; frustrations with the care team; not having the health insurance card could prevent your loved one from being seen by the clinician.

- *Legal risks:* Possible loss of assets or the ability to manage and protect assets; having the ability to pay debts on a timely basis if your loved one's will has to go through probate.

- *Caregiving risks:* Making caregiving more complicated. Caregivers need to be supported so they can spend most of the time caring for your loved one.

Design a strategy: How do I locate the documents and have a way to gather them in an effective time frame? Most documents should be kept, photocopied, and stored in at least two locations: one on-site and one off-site. For example, original documents could be kept in a safe-deposit box and photocopies kept with the power of attorney agent. You can use any of the Cool Tools listed later in this chapter to help with storage options.

My in-laws have put together a three-ring binder with all their pertinent medical documents and medication lists and have diligently kept it current. This was practical and helpful when my father-in-law had a heart attack and his medical information was organized and readily available. Because everything is in one place, it has helped them with following aftercare instructions and comparing changes in medication dosages.

They have also gathered all essential documents, including funeral instructions and a copy of their will, and placed them in a safe location. Family members have been shown the location and given copies of the documents. Their goal was to have everything financial, legal, and health related in one place in the event of an emergency, and it has been a very valuable collection of information. Well done, Grandma and Grandpa.

(Peter Wong)

Execute the plan: If there are additional documents in your loved one's personal situation, add them to your list, locate and copy them, then check it off as completed. You will feel better prepared and have fewer anxieties for your loved one.

Chapter 4 provides information about the important documents you need to gather. Get started on your backup documentation plan by first locating the documents listed in table 11.1. Use the content in the third column as guidance and edit it so that it is current with your resources. For example, your birth certificate may not be in a Wells Fargo safe-deposit box, so change the content to match your location.

Table 11.1. Sample Important Documents Locator Checklist

Document	Photocopied?	Yes/No	Location of Original
Birth certificate			Safe deposit box, Wells Fargo; Carol has key
Driver's license			Wallet
Social Security card			Safe deposit box, Wells Fargo; Carol has key
Medicare/Medicaid card			Dad's is in his wallet; Mom's is in her purse
Insurance card			Dad's is in his wallet; Mom's is in her purse
Mortgage records			Office filing cabinet
Military records			Office filing cabinet
Power of attorney			Office filing cabinet; Attorney Butler's office
Marriage certificate			Safe deposit box, Wells Fargo; Carol has key
Living will, health care proxy, advance directives			Tom and Carol have copy; Attorney Butler's office
Durable power of attorney			Tom and Carol have copy; Attorney Butler
Trust instruments			Tom and Carol have copy; Attorney Butler
Personal health records			Tom and Carol have copy
Credit cards			Tom and Carol have accounts and passwords; Mint.com

After locating and photocopying your original documents, choose a safe but accessible place to keep the copies in the event your power of attorney or a family member needs quick access. Make sure one or two trusted family members or friends are also aware of the location. Creating a list of your document locations now can save both the caregiver and the loved one precious time, money, and future risk.

Backup documentation can be stored in multiple ways. One option is using online storage.

Cool Tools for Online Backup

- *JustCloud:* A free online service, but reviewers say it is difficult to delete folders. Some cost is entailed in expanding the amount of storage.

- *ZipCloud:* Incorporates file versioning, file sharing, automatic backup, and file syncing. $4.95 per month.

- *MyPCBackup:* An industry leader in online backup services with a 9.999999999 percent durability guarantee, meaning that they will lose one file every 10 million years. Free with added features at low monthly costs.

- *Dropbox:* Online storage but not a computer backup site. Files can be accessed from a mobile device, such as an iPad or smartphone. $9.99 per month.

- *SugarSync:* A PCMag.com Editors' Choice and one of the best and simplest services you will find for personal use. $9.99 per month.

Online backup documentation should also include a process to find your documents in the event that the credit card you used to purchase online storage is canceled and the online storage no longer provides access to your account. Problems can also occur if your credit card is reissued for any reason.

Following the Target breach of 2013 that affected more than 100 million credit card customers, many financial institutions issued new cards to protect their customers' accounts from fraud and identity theft. We learned that we were affected when my wife needed to quickly fly to be with her ailing father and the credit card on file with our car rental agency was no longer valid. A new credit card had been issued, but since we had not recently needed a rental car, we hadn't provided the agency with our updated information. In fact, the rental agency required a two-day waiting period for a new card to take effect, but my wife was flying out the next morning. If we had made a list of each corporate service we used that kept our credit card number conveniently on file, we would have contacted each one with our updated information, and my wife would not have needed a taxi to get from the airport to the hospital.

Using online backup is great, but just as one needs a flashlight when the power goes out at home, a manual backup plan is good risk management.

(Peter Wong)

Table 11.2. Sample List: Where to Find Additional Important Original Documents

Documents	Location
Tax returns	Accountant
Birth certificates, Social Security cards, marriage and divorce certificates	Safe deposit box
Insurance, appraisals for valuables	Safe deposit box
Stock, bonds, real estate title, investments	Accountant
Will, copy of durable power of attorney copy, copy of location of safe deposit key with list of contents and names of access authority	Attorney
Letter of instruction not covered by will (personal property for distribution)	Attorney
Estate tax returns	Accountant
Personal business expenses, receipts	Accountant
Checkbook, passports, certificates of deposit	Filing cabinet
Life insurance policies (life, auto, rental, home owner)	Power of attorney
Employee benefit insurance	Filing cabinet

Table 11.2 lists possible locations of additional important documents you will need for you or your loved one. As with table 11.1, delete the location provided and replace with the location you have chosen.

Creating a list of your key contacts and accounts is another important aspect of your documentation plan that will save you many hours as a caregiver. In table 11.3, complete the fields with your own information. For example, in column 1, "Banks," provide key information in column 2.

Key Takeaways

In this chapter, you learned the following:

■ How to create a backup risk management plan for critical information before it is lost.

■ How to create a safe place for your loved ones to find backed-up documentation.

■ How to back up content on your smartphone or handheld device in the event you need to re-create it.

Table 11.3.   Sample List of Important Contacts/Accounts/Information

Contacts	Key Information Needed
Banks	• Name, address, telephone number of each financial institution • Location of passport • Location of checkbooks • Location of bank statement • Location of active loan statements • Beneficiaries on accounts
Attorney	• Name, address, telephone number • Will, trust, power of attorney
Financial planner	• Name, address, telephone number • Account statements • Complete list of beneficiaries
Accountant	• Name, address, telephone number • Tax returns • Documentation of returns
Beneficiary list	Name, address, telephone number

Insurance company and agent	• Name, address, telephone number
	• Type of policy, account number, location:
	    Health
	    Life
	    Auto
	    Home owner
	    Rental
	    Employee
	    Disability
	    Cancer
	    Medicare/Medicaid/Supplemental

Employer pension plan	• Name, address, telephone number
Active credit accounts (banks, mortgage, gas companies, department stores, etc.)	• Name, address, telephone number • Account number and type
Clergy/rabbi	• Name, address, telephone number
E-billing accounts (Netflix, cable, utilities, tuition, etc.)	• Name, address, telephone number • Account number, cycle or statement
Landlord	• Name, address, telephone number

When to Call for Help

Caregivers usually know long before their loved one that it is time to call for backup support, especially if the loved one insists on living an independent life, or aging at home.

In this chapter, calling for help means the following:

- Recognizing signs that you need someone to lift some tasks from your list.

- Knowing when it's time for skilled nursing or adult day care.

- Hiring in-home help.

- Talking to your loved one when you need help.

Signs You Need Help

Families who commit to being a caregiver usually make a promise to provide care for the long haul, whether it's a few months, years, or even decades. For the most part, the rewards of caregiving far outweigh the demands. Disruptions are speed bumps that you learn to glide over. Stress and burnout with long-term care are part of the process. Most of the time, a vacation or sharing the parents with another family member offers relief. You may consider the following:

- Asking others to step in for a while to give you a break

- Wrapping yourself up in something that makes you laugh, such as a comedy playhouse or a funny movie

- Joining a support group where you can confidentially share your frustrations with others

These are not luxuries but necessities.

You, the caregiver, more than any other member of the family, know when you need help. You can feel it deep in your heart. It may feel like guilt or burnout. Other family members see it too but may be afraid to offer anything more than short-term help. If you are the "other family member," we aren't saying you need to take on caregiving because you may not have the time or place to do so. But you do owe the caregiver a promise to be vigilant and step in. Watch for signs and stress that go beyond short-term fixes to become damaging or even hurtful to either the caregiver or the person needing care.

At HelpGuide.org, we found common signs caregivers should watch for that say "it's time to get help":

- You are catching colds and flu much more frequently, or your own health is worsening.

- Your sleep is fitful even though you are in bed for eight hours or more.

- People tell you that you are overreacting to small things.

- You are drinking, smoking, or eating more.

- Even when you get help, you are impatient or irritated with how the person cares for your loved one.

- Family members tell you that you look tired.

- Your loved one complains about the care you are giving.

Signs Your Loved One Needs Outside Help

- The physical layout of your home creating obstacles for mobility

- Frequent incontinence without the ability to clean up after him- or herself

- Complaints of feeling lonely or abandoned when you are away

- Comments that your loved one is despondent or disoriented

- Insensitivity to family needs and consistently expecting to be front and center

- Repeated inappropriate language in spite of your requests to change

- Your body no longer supporting helping your loved one get out of a chair or lie down in bed

When several of these factors make aging at home difficult, it's time for a break; it also may be time to ask for longer-term care.

How to Initiate the Conversation with Your Loved One

In her book *Heart of a Caregiver: Touching Lives with Compassion and Care*, Paula J. Fox says that caregivers look at the world with their hearts. The thought of seeking help from outside sources may be a straightforward business conversation to some but not so straightforward for the caregiver. Anticipate complex emotional dynamics when family and loved one transitions from "aging at home" to "we need some help." You may have experienced some of these dynamics yourself:

- Your loved one may feel guilty for getting sick or being a burden.

- The caregiver may feel you have found fault or blame for not doing enough.

- Family members don't know how they will pay for long-term care.

- The caregiver is not yet ready to let go of the loved one.

- The caregiver wants to reclaim his or her life, and no one can step up to take on caregiving.

Schedule a Family Meeting

Family meetings to discuss outside help require continuous processing for decision making. Make the decision early on whether to include your loved one in the conversation. Our parents would have immediately vetoed any family decisions if they hadn't been a part of the process. Develop an agenda for the family meeting. The following one is provided by SNAPforSeniors:

1. Provide a medical update. A clinical summary from your loved one's recent doctor visit is a good starting point.
2. Share feelings about caregiving and the illness.
3. Describe the daily caregiving needs.
4. Discuss financial concerns, both those as a caregiver and those if your loved one needs a skilled nursing facility.
5. Evaluate options: home health, respite care either with family or a skilled nursing facility, adult day care, long-term care, or hospice.

Eldercare.gov adds these conversation reminders:

- Be patient. Some people may need time to think.

- Don't judge.

- Nothing is set in stone.

- Every attempt at conversation is valuable.

- You don't have to cover everything right now.

- Do you need short-term or longer-term help?

My mother was ninety-three years old and legally blind when she was diagnosed with large granular lymphocytic leukemia, or T-cell leukemia, an aggressive cancer of the blood. If you've been following her story throughout the this book, you also know that she had congestive heart failure, bad knees, and a vow that as long as she was alive, she would keep her commitment to pray for the people she loved.

For years, she promised she would come and live with us, only to corral people in the church to call me with promises that they would care for her if I wouldn't move her from them. Only when I was reconciling her checkbook did I realize she kept a stash of twenty-dollar bills, giving her friends a little something for gas money each time they offered to help.

Lovingly, they took her to church, to the senior center, to the grocery store. Once a week, they took her to her local physician three blocks away to check her hemoglobin.

The plan was that the doctor's office would receive results from the lab the next day, review them to see if they were out of range or had reached "panic value," and then fax results to an oncologist in Kansas City, Missouri, forty-five miles away. The oncologist would then read the results and, if needed, order a blood transfusion at a local community hospital or modify her drugs. Her existence depended on the process: oncologist to neighborhood physician to Mom, who would call a friend to take her to the local community hospital.

The plan worked only if all clinicians opened and read the fax and then called in the order. Sometimes a week or more would go by without the doctors' offices exchanging details.

By the time the two had talked, her red blood count dipped to 5.0 (panic value), and she was deeply fatigued. If she couldn't find or didn't have the strength to call a member of the church to take her to the local hospital, she called 911. EMTs would transport her to the community hospital to stabilize her and then transport her to Liberty Memorial Hospital, a level II trauma center in Liberty, Missouri. Nursing staff there would keep her in the hospital for five to seven days until her platelet level returned to normal range. Then she would be sent home to start the process again.

Each time she crashed, her friends would call me, as I was on their speed dial. Each time, I rerouted my travel plans and caught a flight to her home. Sometimes my brother, Steve, would rush to be at her side. He traveled internationally and wasn't often able to get home on a quick flight.

I was in the business of helping build electronic networks so that physicians and patients could securely exchange health information. I offered to help her local physician transition into electronic records that would help him receive immediate lab results. "Those electronic health records are nothing but government spying into my business," her doctor had said.

It was in pursuit of building the health information technology network that kept my employees and me on the road helping oncologists, nephrologists, and urologists in twenty states migrate medical charts from paper into electronic format. We trained physicians how to electronically order lab tests and receive lab results. I knew that the transition to computers was so time consuming that an old woman's lab results were not top of mind. Mom's lab results were stuck between an overworked oncologist and an old-school doctor. So while we were shepherding doctors into the future, my Momma's health care was caught in the past with doctors' work flow systems dropping her off the charts.

During each of my stays, Mom and I talked about the social and medical benefits of a skilled nursing facility. We both agreed that at ninety-three, she was too independent for a full-time nursing home, but a home health agency would help with daily visits to check her blood pressure and intervene when her hemoglobin started to drop. On one visit, she and I enrolled her in daily home nursing care. We asked about comprehensive background checks for nurses who would be doing the in-home visits. We also asked how the agency monitored their home visit nurses and learned that the agency placed bar codes in the home where the nurse would log in and log out, verifying that she had been at been at the home.

With Mom satisfied with the service, I paid the enrollment fees and coordinated her benefits with Medicare. I also made sure that we secured her home for home nurse visits after the home health supervisor assured Mom that they did comprehensive background checks on each nurse. I felt we had finally reached a middle ground of care.

No sooner had my flight taken off to help a group of oncologists that the supervisor called to say my mom canceled the health plan. That's when I called my brother and said we needed a family meeting with Mom. She either was determined to die in her home or needed full-time skilled nursing care. We wanted to honor Mom's wishes but also ensure she was safe if she wanted to stay at home.

I started reading every article I could find on how to transition parents into a skilled nursing facility, how the conversation would go, and how I should take on parenting my parent. Within a month after canceling home health, she crashed again and was transported to the hospital. This time, Steve and I agreed to transition her directly into a skilled nursing facility where Medicare would pay for the first 100 days. But we needed her buy-in so that she wouldn't walk out of another institution.

"Mom," I said, "you and I both know your body is starting to shut down. You need full-time help."

"Yes, I do," she said. "I need help. But I only have three years of long-term care. What if I live another five years? Who will pay for my care?"

"Momma, let us deal with that. If you stay at home, you won't live another five days."

She was silent, then finally, she said, "Is your brother stateside?"

"Yes, for a few days."

"Then send him first to help me move. He can lift the heavy things. And tell him not to forget my phone. I have people I still need to pray for."

(Carolyn Hartley)

Short-Term Help

Respite care is short-term care provided in a nursing home, hospice inpatient, or hospital, allowing the caregiver time to rest or take some time off. A break for you may also mean an opportunity for your loved one to get oriented to a community setting. Your loved one also may need convalescent care following surgery.

The most common question caregivers ask is not whether they deserve a break but how they will pay for services. Medicare.gov offers guidance on benefits for many services, including respite care and where to find a location that accepts Medicare/Medicaid. Your loved one will need Medicare Part A (Hospital Insurance) coverage services. This covers inpatient hospital stays, hospice care, home health care, and care in a skilled nursing facility. A robust search engine will check to see if respite care is covered and for how many days.

We also like the depth of information and guidance available at Eldercare.gov, a public service of the Administration on Aging. This is a nationwide service that will connect you with Area Agencies on Aging. These services are designed primarily to help seniors age in their homes.

If you are the caregiver for a mentally or physically disabled young adult, you may find help with another resource. In 2009, the U.S. Congress authorized the Lifespan Respite Care Program. These are "coordinated systems of accessible, community-based respite care services for caregivers of children and adults of all ages with special needs."

Group homes for the disabled provide housing and meals. Most also provide activities for their residents and often help them find employment. Consult the Administration for Community Living, an agency within the U.S. Department of Health and Human Services, to learn more about community living arrangements, such as group homes, and whether it is a good fit for your loved one. You can also search for community or group homes in your area by putting "community living services" plus your ZIP code into a search engine. We recommend you also search for quality ratings from the Administration for Community Living. Public reviews posted online are a source of good information, but then ask for the following if you are considering a group home:

- Accreditation and accrediting agencies

- Sources of public and private funding

- Summary report of most recent inspection

- Alliance with other organizations that offer services, such as the following:

  - Rehabilitation

  - Mobility and transportation

  - Employment training and help

  - Benefits checkup (e.g., with the National Council on Aging), used to screen for benefits programs for seniors with limited income and resources

  - Personal safety training with a focus on preventing bullying and abuse (Our favorite for kids of all ages is Kidpower, a nonprofit California-based organization that offers training in person or at long distance.)

How to Find a Long-Term Care Facility

Choosing a long-term care facility may be relatively easy for you if you live in a smaller community and the long-term care facility near your home consistently receives high marks from inspectors. While both of us have been involved in finding skilled nursing facilities for family members (also called long-term care, or nursing homes), it is our goal not to reinvent the search process but rather to show you tools developed by many before us. We provide those in the Cool Tools section.

We also regularly made our own physical inspections and include that list in table 12.1. These are things we never thought to ask until it happened to our family members. Medicare.gov also posts inspection criteria for families seeking help from long-term care facilities.

Table 12.1. On-Site Checklist for Long-Term Care Facilities

Category	What to Look For	What We Found	Your Findings
Clothing	Is your loved one wearing someone else's clothes? Who does your loved one's laundry?	We purchased white socks by the dozen every six months and wrote his name on each pair. Within two months, he was wearing worn socks with holes and someone else's shirts. We did see other men wearing his socks.	
Pressure sores	Roll back the covers and lift your loved one's clothes and check around his or her waist, hips, back, and legs.	We often found pressure sores (also called bedsores) on my father's hips and reported them to his physician. After the aides realized we checked regularly, my father ceased to have pressure sores.	
Nutrition	Can your loved one feed him- or herself? Does the facility hire a nutritionist?	My father wore false teeth, but during a housecleaning, they were lost or destroyed. Finally, the nutritionist transitioned him to a soft diet.	
Bathing	Who bathes your loved one?	Dignity was our primary concern. We found my father to be bathed and showered at least every other day by a male aide.	
Odors	Do rooms smell of feces?	We found that my father's room generally was clean and well attended.	
Daily activities	Does your loved one receive daily exercise, as appropriate?	My father would watch *Animal Planet* 24/7/365 if they let him. The nurses engaged him in daily activities to relieve soreness in his joints.	

Category	What to Look For	What We Found	Your Findings
Roommate	In a semiprivate room, are the roommate's family respectful of your loved one's health and personal items?	During one of our inspections, we found the roommate's family member smoking in the room and rummaging through my father's closet. We confronted him immediately and also reported the incident to Medicare.gov as well as to the safety officer.	

When to Call Hospice

"Hospice has been called in" means that the health care team is no longer focusing on finding a cure but is now focused on comfort, equipment, medications, and symptom management for the patient and also for the family. It also may mean bereavement counseling, but that is not the immediate goal. Talk with your doctor if you're thinking about getting treatment to cure your illness. As a hospice patient, you always have the right to stop hospice care at any time.

When you call in hospice, you immediately begin lowering your health costs. Just as important, you also begin engaging the family in logical and progressive next steps.

Your physician is the person to order hospice. You may initiate the conversation by calling hospice for information to request a consultation and find out if your loved one qualifies for hospice care. Generally, hospice is paid by Medicare for six months, but your hospice physician can recertify you for another six-month period if the illness is terminal.

All care that you receive in managing a terminal illness must be given by or arranged by the hospice team. You can still see your regular doctor if you've chosen him or her to be the attending medical professional who helps supervise hospice care.

Medicare doesn't cover room and board if you get hospice care in your home or if you live in a nursing home or a hospice inpatient facility. Medicare will, however, cover a short-term inpatient or respite care service that hospice arranges. You may have to pay a small copayment for the respite stay. Coordinate emergency room care, inpatient facility care, or ambulance transports with hospice to avoid having to pay out of pocket for these costs.

Palliative care is similar to hospice care. The most significant difference is that hospice reimbursement requires that an individual be diagnosed as terminally ill.

Palliative care, often offered in hospitals, skilled nursing facilities, and the home, involves medications, equipment, or prescription drugs. You do not need to be diagnosed with a terminal illness to receive palliative care.

Who's eligible for hospice? You are eligible for hospice under these conditions:

- You're eligible for Medicare Part A (Hospital Insurance).

- Your doctor certifies that you're terminally ill and are expected to have six months or less to live.

- You accept palliative care (for comfort) instead of care to cure your illness.

- You sign a statement choosing hospice care instead of routine Medicare-covered benefits for your terminal illness.

In a Medicare-approved hospice facility, nurse practitioners can serve in place of an attending physician if the doctor first certifies the illness. You may be charged a minimal copayment of no more than $5 for each prescription drug and other similar products for pain relief and symptom control while you're at home.

Cool Tools

Additional tools for care conversations are available at these websites:

- Hospicedirectory.org

- Hospicenet.org

- CareConversations.org

- PBS: "Starting the Conversation About Long Term Care: 10 Things You Should Know"

- ElderCare.gov, "Let's Talk"

Tips and resources from Medicare include the following:

- What will Medicare cover?

- What should every caregiver know about Medicare?

- When to call hospice

Key Takeaways

In this chapter, you learned the following:

- Asking for help can be a difficult task for caregivers. Family members should assist by looking for signs that the caregiver is stressed or getting burned out.

- Help can be short-term respite care, long-term skilled nursing, or home health for seniors aging at home.

- When selecting a facility, consult Medicare.gov and similar sources that offer findings from quality inspections.

- Include all family members in conversations when you need help.

Section 3

DEALING WITH DEATH

Dealing with death is "heart work." Caregivers are the ones who see it first. Caregivers often view death as a blessing, bringing their loved one to a closer presence with God. They also see death as the leading cause of self-imposed guilt, wondering what they could have done to have made their loved one's life more comfortable.

Having had the privilege and a distinct honor to be present at passing, we find death to be a comforting blend of science, medicine, and spiritual connectedness. Death is a full-blown heart makeover, one that uses joy, relief, sorrow, compassion, and prayer to cut, paste, and spin each of us into a new person.

If you are called to be at the bedside, you are one lucky person. Dying is the most common outcome of caregiving. Having been deeply honored to be involved in the process ourselves, we share with dignity the lessons learned and brilliant guidance we received from our counselors.

13 Know When to Say Good-Bye

When it was our turn to say good-bye to family and friends, we talked to ministers, hospice nurses, authors, and health care professionals. We said a whole lot of prayers asking for love to fill the black hole in our hearts. Those conversations are so much easier to write about today than it was to manage then.

We found that it helped to lean a little on medical and psychology journals and prayers, and we listened to the training provided by hospice nurses. Straight talk was the best therapy. We hope that what we learned will help you too.

In this chapter, we provide you with guidance on the following:

- How you can help your loved one "die well."

- What dying people want to hear from their loved ones.

- Signs the body gives that say death is near.

- What to do when death finally comes.

- How to say good-bye.

You Can Help Your Loved One Die Well

Jewish wisdom provides a total framework around humanity in which the family and community consider a "dying person" to be fully living in every respect. This wisdom requires a complete person to be in human relations even unto death without depriving the dying person of joy. In some Asian cultures, telling a person he or she is dying is considered unnecessary cruelty. Some Hispanic and African American families want the physician to keep their loved one alive, no matter how ill they are, while European communities believe that life-prolonging measures should be discontinued. Judaism shields mourners from being overwhelmed by the process of saying good-bye. The community of family and friends shares the experience together, helping the dying person as well as those left behind to be embraced. You should plan to talk about your culture's approach to dying with your physician. In the United States, though, dying is treated as if it is a separate realm of existence, often leaving us with guilt: "Why didn't the nurse or doctor get here earlier?" or "If you had performed these tests a year ago, my mother would not have died."

The bioethics of dying in the United States is a legal process designed for white, middle-class families with a Western philosophical tradition. In the past two decades, we have turned the process of dying over to medical professionals, most of whom acknowledge that when business processes are put in place, dying can be more peaceful. Hospitals require advance directives as part of the official medical chart. Without an advance directive, the state will step in and impose state requirements on how your loved one's passing will be handled. Some cultures don't want legal documents to determine how long to prolong life.

Alex Kodiath, MD, says in his book *Elder Care: Precious Presence* that people trying to avoid death send their loved ones to the hospital. "While the family clings to hope that the loved one can be saved, it ultimately serves only to aggravate the patient's last moments. Families feel they must do something." Dr. Kodiath, a physician who works in long-term care, says your greatest gift may be your presence of grace. Dying well is a complex and overwhelming process.

Pain is most likely very present. Patients receiving palliative care may be taking multiple drugs to ease the pain. Often these analgesic measures result in side effects, from hallucinations and outbursts to high sensitivity to touch. Some patients want to be cognizant of everything that is happening around them, while others simply want to go numb and stop the pain. Some cultures set aside time for rituals or spiritual consultation, ensuring that the believer's pathway has been blessed for ascent into heaven. Others may burn incense to invite the presence of ancestors to carry the loved one to his or her new home. Dr. Reggie Anderson writes in his book *Appointments with Heaven* that people who believe in heaven often say they see family members and begin talking to them.

These rituals or spiritual gatherings are part of the dignity you are offering your loved one, giving them "permission to die." Hearing is the last sense to go, so even if your loved one is in a coma, assume everything you say can be heard.

What Dying People Want to Hear
Talk about your loved one as if he or she is still in the room. Lie next to the person in bed or hold hands to say parting words. If it's possible, let them feel your

warm breath against their neck. Familiar and soft music may offer additional comfort.

Do not judge others if they cannot be in the room. Not everyone can do this, but do not let them control your decision to be present. Tell your reluctant spouse or family member that it is okay to not be present but that you need to be here in the room.

Find a way to tell your loved one the five things they want to hear most:

1. You will take care of the things he or she was responsible for. For example, you might say the following:
    a. "I am so glad you walked me through your house maintenance plan. Remember, we built a book, and it has all the people you rely on to keep the yard looking the way you want it."
    b. "You showed me how to be a great leader. It will take some time for me to step into your shoes, but you set such a great example for me. I can take it from here."
2. Your children and your spouse will be okay:
    a. "Our children will be sad for a while, but they will be okay."
    b. "We will survive. We will be okay because of your great work."
    c. "We will be loving your children and taking care of them. You have a large extended family."
3. Talk about how your loved one will be remembered:
    a. Say thank you for a wonderful life.
    b. Praise him or her for what coworkers and friends have said about him or her.
    c. Remind him or her of the beautiful house he or she built for you and how safe you feel.
    d. Move something to another place and say, "Every time I see that picture of you and me, I will remember how much you loved me."
    e. "I can see your likeness in your children's eyes; what a blessing to others."
4. If you suspect that your loved one needs any forgiveness, offer it now. You may have forgotten all about any transgressions, but as people near passing, they remember things they should have done differently or with more compassion. They may experience short-term memory loss, but long-term memory, such as the line you said at the seventh-grade musical, is alive and well.

For the last five years of my mother's life, she always ended every phone call with "I love you. Please forgive me for not standing up for you when you were young."

My grandfather was sixty-four years old when my father was born in 1918, the ninth child born to a family of Canadian fishermen. I'm quite sure my father was not an easy child, having seven sisters, none of whom wanted to touch a fish, but each sister was eager for my dad to grow up and take over the business. Oddly, my father became a fisher of men and went into the ministry. Until he transitioned into education for disabled children, he parented like his father. Rough, ready, shipshape. Tough.

We would tell my mother, "Mom, that's in the past. We have found our own paths of healing, and we forgave you and Dad long ago."

Sometimes I would add, "Mom, this is still bothering you. Please talk through this guilt with someone who can help you find relief."

"I do. I talk to God every day."

Somehow God's and our forgiveness hadn't found its way into her heart because we'd hear it again the next call.

After so many flights home to be at her side each time her hemoglobin dropped below 6.0, I finally understood what she wanted. I crawled beside her in bed and held her hand. We listened to an audiotape about Grace and Forgiveness from Dr. James Dobson. My mother was a musician who performed in churches across the country, so we also listened to "Israel" by the Gaither Vocal Band. I wanted to pour grace and love into her heart as much as I could while lying at her side.

I didn't think it was my place to forgive her. She had been a magnificent mom. I loved and cherished her deeply. But as children, when Dad took off his belt, she knelt at the foot of the bed and prayed that her children would not feel the pain rather than standing up to him and telling him to stop.

The one time she did stand up to him, my dad moved out of the house for a week, leaving her alone with four children. We never had so much fun. But for my mom, it was a living hell. He promised he could never be married to a disobedient wife, so she asked for forgiveness, and he moved back in. Things started to get better between them and between Dad and us. My mom set aside her brilliant independent mind to be a good wife and mother.

The hardest words I ever said to her finally came out: "Mom. I forgive you. I forgive you for not taking a sledgehammer to Dad when we were children. I forgive you for not offering yourself as a sacrifice when Dad started beating us. But I thank you most for giving us the power to forgive. Today, even when we know it isn't our fault, we forgive, and that is so much more powerful than getting even. Your children are successful today because Dad taught us duty, but you taught us grace."

(Carolyn Hartley)

5. Tell your loved one how he or she made a difference. Praise your loved one for the gifts he or she brought into your life.
   a. Material wealth, such as a comfortable home or a new car
   b. Family events, such as getting kids through college, family vacations, or playing baseball in the backyard
   c. Spiritual presence and participation in faith activities
   d. Community leadership or volunteer work
   e. Comments from coworkers about what your loved one has done
   f. Comments of being a role model, an example, or a faithful friend to others
   g. Comments of being a courageous and faithful father
   h. Comments of being a loving and caring mother and spouse

"Dying people have the uncanny ability to choose the moment of death, and it's not uncommon for them to spare those they love the most or feel protective of by waiting until those people leave the room," says Maggie Callanan, Massachusetts hospice nurse and the author of *Final Journeys: A Practical Guide for Bringing Care and Comfort at the End of Life*, who has witnessed more than 2,000 deaths. She advises families not to wait until the last breath to tell your loved one what you really wanted them to know.

Clinical Signs the Body Gives That Say Death Is Near

Science and the medical process can be a tremendous death-processing mechanism. Most of us are not trained to manage the end-of-life events that happen to the body. So, if you are squeamish, you should move on to our section on hospice. However, if you are watching for signs, rely first on medical advice. The following list is intended to support guidance offered by your family physician or palliative care doctors. Most of these recommendations come from Ira Byock, MD, a well-known palliative care physician and author of *Dying Well* and *The Best Care Possible*. Dr.

Byock advocates for a natural dying process and also indicates that the following processes will be different with patients connected to life support:

1. *Loss of appetite:* Your loved one may decline meals or liquids or may request only bland foods that are easily digested. If your loved one requests a favorite food, share in the joy of eating it together. (Make mine lemon meringue pie with chocolate kisses on the side.) Some medications make it difficult to swallow. If swallowing is a problem, your hospice physician can administer some pain medications through a suppository, by injection or infusion, or by placing a patch on the skin. To manage fluid intake, offer a popsicle, ice chips, or sips of water. Dip a clean washcloth into cool water to moisten the lips or use a balm to keep the lips from cracking.

2. *Excessive fatigue and sleeping:* Allow your loved one to sleep without abruptly awakening or shaking to be alert.

> I flew to be with my sister on several occasions during the 100 days after she was diagnosed with cancer. The last time I arrived at her home before she passed, she had slipped into a coma. The family had gathered, and a hospice nurse was always close by. We knew the end was close. I wanted more than anything for Kath to wake up and say, "I love you." Her husband said, "Kathy, Carolyn just arrived. She's here with us now." Immediately my sister's breathing pattern changed as she took deep breaths trying to awaken herself. I said, "I love you too, my seester," our secret code from childhood. She was calm and relaxed in a bed facing the garden she had so tenderly built. Then I asked the family's permission before climbing into bed beside her to stroke her cheek.
> (Carolyn Hartley)

3. *Increased physical weakness:* Your loved one may not be able to sit up in bed or may experience myoclonic jerking, or sudden muscle twitches or jerks from patients taking opioids for pain relief. Maintain focus on your loved one's comfort and assume that your loved one can still hear everything you say.

4. *Disorientation or mental confusion:* Your loved one may not be aware of where he or she is or who else is in the room. As the caregiver, you may need to explain this to family members who come to say good-bye and hope to be recognized. Your loved one may wave to someone they see in the ceiling or say nonsensical things. Remain calm, acknowledge that he

or she is seeing someone, and identify yourself when you approach. Touch the person's feet first, then slowly move your hand up the legs so that your loved one can connect with your presence.

5. *Urination changes*: As your loved one takes in less fluid, the body will become more dehydrated, resulting in a state of ketosis. During ketosis, the body uses fat and muscle as a fuel source, producing a state of well-being and peaceful euphoria. With fluid cutback, the blood pressure will drop, and kidneys begin to fail. Blood toxins make the dying process more peaceful. Urine may be brownish, reddish, or tea colored. As the caregiver, you should ask close family members to maintain a twenty-four-hour vigil with three- to four-hour intervals and respond to the loved one's needs. The schedule may last three to seven days.

6. *Labored breathing:* Cheyne-Stokes respiration might be heard: a loud, deep inhalation, followed by a pause of not breathing or apnea for five to sixty seconds, after which a loud deep breath begins the process again. You will be more prepared for this as the caregiver, but the breathing (often gurgling) sounds may alarm listeners. Slightly elevate your loved one's head or turn the body sideways. Remember to moisturize the lips with balm or petroleum jelly.

7. *Swollen extremities:* As the heart slows its beating process, body fluid may accumulate, forming pools around the feet, hands, or face. This is a natural part of the dying process. Don't provide any diuretics. This is a natural process. However, your physician may prescribe Lasix to reduce bloating.

8. *Coolness in fingers and toes:* As the blood pumps even less into the periphery of the body, the fingers and toes become notably colder. Nail beds are likely to turn bluish. If your loved one complains of being cold, put a blanket over his or her torso.

9. *Loss of bowel or bladder control:* To most caregivers, this is just another day in the life of a caregiver. A hospice worker may recommend a catheter but not in the final hours. Add a bed pad when you are changing the sheets.

10. *Mottled veins:* Mottled veins look like they are close to protruding through the skin, similar to varicose veins, but now they are in the feet, legs, and arms. This is the result of reduced blood flow and a sign that death is at hand.

When Kathy died, her adult children, her husband, hospice nurse, and I were in the room talking softly about family when Stan looked over at her and said, "She's gone."

It was just like Kath, to protect us and slip away quietly. Holding hands, we said the Lord's Prayer together. Each person whispered to her and kissed her. Then the women gathered in the most remarkable ceremony, rubbing hyssop and juniper berry oils on her body. Someone would hum a tune now and then, but mostly we worshipped her body as we clothed her in essential oils. These oils not only took away our sorrowful energy but also acted to purify the room, uplift spirits, and begin the process of healing with positive energy. It also gave us something to do with our hands as we collectively passed passion and love into her earthly body, all the while blessing us with aromatherapy.

When her husband and children agreed it was time, the hospice nurse called the funeral home to come and take her body. As long as I live, I will encourage others to participate in this gracious and womanly tribute.

(Carolyn Hartley)

Cool Tools

- *When Should You Call in Hospice?* This tool, provided by PalliativeDoctors. org, provides a few answers to the most commonly asked hospice questions. If your doctor determines that your loved one has less than six months to live, you are likely to find insurance from Medicare, Medicaid, and your own insurance. Our favorite quote on this page is, "Hospice is not about giving up. It's about giving you comfort, control, dignity and quality of life."

- *How to Find a Hospice near You:* Mentioned in chapter 12, we found two reputable sites worthy of your inquiries: HospiceDirectory.org and Hospicenet.org. Caregivers who find themselves repeating the caregiving process may choose to participate in a more career-oriented way. If this is the case for you, consult Hospicefoundation.org. All these websites are reliable and advertisement free and have a lot of information to help you through end-of-life issues. These websites will direct you to quality articles written by physicians and patient families as well as where to find support groups after your loved one passes. Most hospice facilities will check on family members for twelve to fifteen months after the funeral to be sure you have a support group helping you through the grieving process.

- *Say Good-bye to Caregiver Guilt:* No matter how much you do, caregivers frequently believe that they could have managed life differently for their loved one. "Guilt can be destructive," says Dr. Alexis Anderson in her blog for the Eldercare Sacramento. The ten tips provided here will help you process your feelings and heal from the inside out.

- *Essential Oils for Holistic Aromatherapy:* The National Association for Holistic Aromatherapy provides a list of the most commonly used oils for relieving stress, strengthening the immune system, and healing a wound.

- *Caring.com:* This website focuses on those who provide care. While we mention them throughout this book, it's worth mentioning them again.

Key Takeaways

In this chapter, you learned the following:

- When it's time to call in a palliative care provider, such as hospice.

- The family must shift from a focus on the disease to a focus on the patient's comfort.

- The patient's comfort is top of mind in all medicines and activities.

- There are some drugs you can administer; others can be given only by a hospice clinical staff member.

- Depending on your loved one's condition, hospice will show you how to give gentle back rubs, foot massages, or scalp massages.

- The clinical staff will tell you what to watch for, letting you know when to call friends and family to pay final respects.

- Tell your loved one the five things he or she most wants to hear.

- As the loved one's caregiver, take the lead informing friends and family, as appropriate, on how to deal with the dying process.

14 | Planning the Funeral

Caregivers frequently say their skills are never put to the test more than when their loved one passes away. Relief, frustration, anxiety over the future, new processes, medical bills, and much more begin churning day and night. Friends and family help caregivers go into "event-planning mode," celebrating the life of the family or friend. Often, the funeral home director is the one who takes over the actual plans, guiding the family through decisions, many of which can be costly if not defined prior to the funeral. As with most events, parts of the funeral will go well, and other things will be rough, so a plan will help direct the dazed and comforted into a focused direction.

Funerals require a multitude of decisions in a very short amount of time. This chapter focuses on the following:

- Funerals and event planning.

- Step-by-step instructions that can save you and the family time, money, and missteps.

- Tips to manage family members who disagree with the deceased's wishes.

Funerals and Memorials Are Events

You've just suffered through a life-altering experience through the enormous loss of a family member. Now the family looks to you to continue your caregiving leadership by putting on your event-planning hat.

Funerals are highly emotional events that too often take place with very little time for planning. Emotional purchases usually result in higher costs. Consider yourself fortunate if you and your loved one have preplanned the funeral, as it is one of the greatest acts of love a dying person can offer to his or her caregiver and family.

Most loved ones will consider favorite songs they would like played at the funeral. Some songs offer comfort or rejoice in the hereafter. Songs are but a small part of funeral planning, but thinking through music is uplifting to loved ones who want to leave behind a message of hope and courage. Sometimes music is all the loved one can get through.

Your job as the funeral planner is to quickly pull together family resources, files, pictures, and calendars. Together, you will express the family's desire for an event that symbolizes your loved one's character, impact on others' lives, and memories you want others to remember.

Calloused as it may seem, caregivers need to slip away during the last few days of the loved one's life and go through funeral plans. Your meeting with the funeral director may seem like an emotional transaction, but to the funeral home it's a business transaction. Yes, the staff know that you are grieving and will offer comfort, but they are in the business of managing death and performing funerals.

We recommend that you talk through your plans with a business friend before you meet with the funeral home. It's your turn to have an advocate. At any time during the on-site planning meeting, you can ask to take a break and think things through. In fact, we encourage this. In the next section, we help you "suit up" for the business discussion.

Preplan for the Funeral Director Meeting

1. *Call your clergy.*
   a. Allow time for this conversation.
   b. Clergy have done a lot more funerals than most of us and can provide calming guidance.
   c. If you are not a member of a faith community, hospice may help connect you with a counselor.
2. *What funeral home has been selected?*
   a. Is it centrally located with enough room for parking?
   b. Do you have a personal relationship with the owners?
   c. Is there a prepaid plan?
3. *What does your loved one want to do with the remains?*
   a. Buried, cremated, or offered to science?
      i. Burial generally requires a casket and a cemetery.
      ii. Cremation does not require a casket or cemetery, but you will likely want to purchase an urn. These can run into the thousands of dollars, so shop around. You are not required to use the funeral home's urn

selection. Extended family members may request a small portion of the ashes. If this meets with your family's approval, ask them to pay for their own miniature urns. If not, respond consistently to all requests.

    iii. Donating the whole body to science is done prior to death. Many states also require that this be a clause in the individual's last will and testament. Complete an online search using the key words "willed body program" plus your city and state to determine the process for this donation.

  b. Organ donors are still buried.

    i. If your loved one is an organ donor, go to Organdonor.gov to learn more about the process.

    ii. Most successful organ donations come from victims of severe head trauma, a brain aneurism, or stroke and must be pronounced brain dead (not in a coma) by a licensed neurologist. Organ donations do not require a will but do require your loved one to have preregistered to be a donor, for example, through a state driver's licensing agency. If there is no documentation, the hospital must obtain written approval from next of kin.

4. *Where is the cemetery?*

  a. Are there restrictions on the types of monuments or memorials?

  b. Is there a family plot?

  c. Is your loved one a veteran? All veterans are entitled to a free burial in a national cemetery and a grave marker. For more information, go to the National Cemetery Administration of the Veterans Administration.

5. *What are the costs?*

  a. The Federal Trade Commission (FTC) Funeral Rule went into effect in 1984. This rule set in place national guidelines to protect funeral consumers from fraud and deception and also set in place how funeral homes could sell their goods and services. Funeral homes with a website provide a general price list. We found a generic consumer-friendly list guide from Funerals.org that provides a seventeen-page document filled with definitions, common errors, low and high prices, and key words that indicate hidden costs. It's a great read if you have time and could potentially save you thousands of dollars. The FTC also provides a list of costs worksheet to help you calculate the estimated funeral services cost from the funeral home and cemetery. A reprint of this worksheet is provided in Cool Tools.

b. The FTC's list represents funeral home costs only. We've added costs for you to include in your budget in the same worksheet.

c. Who is paying?

   i. If your loved one prepaid funeral costs, there should be a folder in your loved one's files that itemize what has been prepaid. Take this with you to visit with the funeral director. This is really important, as we have heard stories from families who paid for a funeral, only to discover months later that the funeral had been prepaid elsewhere.

   ii. Generally, the person who held durable power of attorney pays funeral costs, but upon death it is the executor trustee who has authority to pay for funeral bills. For example, the executor trustee is a joint owner of the loved one's savings account intended to cover funeral costs. Consult chapters 4 and 15 on how to ensure that the trustee is listed on the loved one's bank accounts.

   iii. If your loved one does not have a savings account, the executor trustee (probably you, the caregiver) should reimburse yourself when you process and receive death benefits.

   iv. Keep all receipts and track expenses in a spreadsheet. You will need to include these costs in the loved one's final tax report. Receipts include the following:

- Executor trustee's travel costs
- Durable goods donations, such as clothing, furniture, and appliances
- Cost of flowers
- Bulletins for the service
- Funeral home's expenses
- Clergy donations, generally around $100
- Musicians donations, generally around $75 to $100
- Church maintenance fees
- Hairdresser if you want a personal touch
- Military color guard, if applicable

d. Prepare items to be brought to the funeral home.

   i. The funeral director should give you a list. Our list changes every time, but generally it includes these items:

- Clothing for the deceased to wear in the casket
- Information about the deceased, including the following:
  Social Security number
  Birth date, city, county, and state

Marital status

Veterans discharge papers or claim number

- Deceased parents' names, including mother's maiden name
- Details about the deceased's education
- A recent photo
- Cemetery lot information
- Name of clergy performing the funeral
- Names of pallbearers and honorary pallbearers, such as grand-children
- Obituary (Most funeral homes will post the obituary at no charge in up to three newspapers. They will have a word count, so plan on extra charges if the obit exceeds word counts and if you want more newspapers notified.)
- Know how many death certificates you need (Ask for at least ten notarized copies. Some families ask for fifteen. You will need an original notarized copy for each death benefit you file. It's much easier and less expensive to get them now than later.)

6. *The FTC Funeral Rule applies to funeral homes supporting families of all faiths.* For example, families of the Jewish faith often bury the loved one within twenty-four hours of death and then enter a seven-day period of mourning. The first few days of mourning are reserved for family. Friends usually wait until at least the third day to visit. Do not make a call on the Sabbath (Friday afternoon until after dark on Saturday). Plan to visit the family in the evening or on Sunday of the week after the death.

My mother gave me the greatest gift of all before she died. She had asked me several times to go with her to the funeral home and help her pick out a casket. I was squeamish about that, knowing I should, until finally I put on my big-girl face and agreed to a time and date. I picked Mom up in my car and drove to the funeral home. While we were still in the parking lot, I said a prayer not only to ask for guidance but also to acknowledge the 800-pound gorilla sitting between us. We were here to pick out a casket. After that, things got kind of funny.

The funeral director took us into the showroom and then left us alone to shop. This was a shopping trip? It went like this.

"Carolyn, I'd like to wear my pink dress, but I'm a little overweight right now, so could you ask the funeral director not to fill me with so much embalming fluid."

That set the stage. This was going to be real and straight-up talk.

"Okay." I took out my notepad and started writing.

"What color do you think the liner should be, white or black?" Mom asked.

"I think white satin would look better with your pink dress."

"And what casket do you think we should pick? I'll be lying next to Dad, and I don't think I should show him up by having a nicer resting place than him."

"I think you should," I said.

That's when we found the casket named "pearl." My mom's name was Pearl. Creeee-py! "That's the one, Mom," I said.

"Write that one down." she said.

"I don't think I'll forget."

"Now what about the pillow?" Mom asked. "I don't want a pillow under my head. That would give me a headache."

"Mom, you're not going to be feeling anything."

"Yes, but the pillow will show my double chin."

I pulled out my notepad. "No double chin."

"How about if we put the pillow at my side, sort of angled up like this? With a cross of roses."

Scribble, scribble on my notepad.

"Call my friend Eileen and tell her to do my hair. I've seen how they do hair here. It's so phony."

"Got it."

"Be sure they give me eyebrows and pink lipstick."

Eyebrows, I wrote. Lipstick—pink.

"And do you see this pullout drawer?" She tugged on a drawer inside the casket. "Please ask all of the grandkids to write me a note so I'll remember to pray for them in heaven."

That's when I lost it. Thank goodness for my mom's sense of humor because she lost it too. The scene was just too incredibly insane to cry, so we cried and laughed at the same time until the funeral director asked if we needed help.

"Yes, we need help!" I said. "My mother's dying, but she's wisecracking with casket stories."

Then my mom did the most amazing thing. She pulled out her checkbook and paid for everything on the spot. When she died, I did not have to worry about clothes or cost or colors. She took care of it all.

(Carolyn Hartley)

Day of the Meeting

Count on the funeral home to provide you with a general price list for services. Some funeral homes provide this online if they have a website. If possible, look at the list prior to your meeting.

Ask family members to help you gather items for your meeting at least several hours before your scheduled appointment. When you arrive, plan to listen first to the funeral director. He or she is experienced in walking you through the details, and this will give you time to regain composure. The director will get to the general price list in due time. This is when you pull out your list and compare prices. Lean on your business advocate to help with decision making.

We offer here our lessons learned from being the bereaved business advocate:

- Most funeral homes set a time for visitation to comply with state laws and their schedules. Be sure visitation times are compatible with your family's plans as well.

- Ask if you can set up a memorial table outside the viewing room and when you can get into the funeral home to set this up. Find out if they have a table or if you need to bring your own.

- Ask if the family can have private time together before guests start arriving.

- Ask the funeral director to clearly walk through all the plans for the day of visitation and the day of the funeral.

- Ask about who will notify the pallbearers what to do. The funeral director should take care of this.

When People Offer to Help

Nearly all etiquette books say close friends and family should come to the house as soon as they learn of your loved one's passing. They should stay for ten to fifteen minutes unless you ask them to stay longer. During this time, people nearly always ask, "Please let me know what I can do to help." Decide now to accept help but also provide a checklist like the one in table 14.1.

Faith communities with a bereavement committee will offer to sponsor a lunch or dinner after the internment. Accept this help, but you will need a coordinator. We added that to the list as well.

Tasks That Must Be Handled by the Family

Good for you if friends and loved ones take on a task or bring food to help you through the next few days. But there are some tasks that need to be done by the

Table 14.1. Volunteer Checklist

Message at the top: Our family thanks you for your kindness and support, especially during the next few days. If there is a task below you wish to manage, we offer our most heartfelt thanks for your gifts.

(Suggested) Tasks	Volunteer and Phone Number	Day 2	Day 3	Day 4	Day 5	Day 6	Day 7
Build a page on our website for people to access information about <name's> funeral.							
Create a call tree to notify friends and family of your loved one's passing.							
Build a list of hotels, car rental agencies, addresses, and phone numbers. Post on website and make twenty-five hard copies for people as they stop by.							
Coordinate food supply for the next five days. Keep a list of friends who volunteered to bring food.							
Create three maps: (1) from our home to the funeral home, (2) from the funeral home to the cemetery, and (3) from the cemetery to the church or synagogue for a luncheon. Include addresses for each.							

(Suggested) Tasks	Volunteer and Phone Number	Day 2	Day 3	Day 4	Day 5	Day 6	Day 7
Gather pictures and personal items for a memorial table.							
Help pull together a memorial video for the funeral service.							
Pick up family members from the airport.							
Call volunteers and remind them of their task.							
Decide on a charity you'd like to receive donations in your loved one's honor.							
Answer the door or phone for friends and family as they arrive at the house.							
Keep a record of visitors and food and flower deliveries for thank-you notes.							
Arrange for child care as needed.							
Disburse flowers after the funeral.							
Call maid service to clean the house.							
Help elderly friends and family get in and out of cars.							

Table 14.2.   Family-Only Postfuneral Tasks

Task	Family Member	When	Status
Immediately ensure you have cash on hand, as the bank will freeze any accounts where the deceased was the sole owner.	Executor trustee	Just prior to death, if you have time	
Select pallbearers.	Executor trustee	Day 2 after death	
Review duration of automatic deposits following the death. Some retirement plans continue to issue payments for thirty or sixty days after death, depending on the policy.	Executor trustee	Seven to ten days	
Obtain the will and make copies of all pages that establish you as the executor trustee and the notarized signature page. You will likely need twenty copies.		Seven to ten days	
Build a chart of all insurance policies, retirement plans, investments, credit unions, military accounts, bank accounts, and so on. Check on continued income from all sources. These are discussed in chapter 15.	Financial planner, lawyer, or executor Trustee	Seven to ten days	
Consult credit cards. Ask for additional time due to death if applicable. You will need to provide documentation.	Executor trustee	Seven to ten days	
Pay all debts to utility companies.		Seven to ten days	
Notify post office where to send mail if your loved one was living alone.		Seven to ten days	
Communicate these steps with family to better manage questions down the road.		Continuous	

executor trustee and family. Some need to be done immediately. Others can wait for seven to ten days. Table 14.2 provides a list of family-specific tasks.

Writing the Memorial (Obituary)

Many funeral homes will write the obituary for you and send it to a few newspapers. But some families want to write the obituary themselves. We chose to write these ourselves, and it served as a family bonding exercise where we began telling stories about the deceased. An outline for the obituary is provided in table 14.3.

Table 14.3.   Obituary Outline

Sample Phrases	Details to Collect	Notes
Mary Elizabeth Swanson, MD, went to be with her Lord on <date>.	Name: first, middle, last Maiden name	
	Titles (Jr., III, MD, etc.)	
	Include a photo.	
She was born on <month, year> to <name of parents>.	Birthplace and month and year of birth	
	Parents' names	
She lived in <place>.	List cities and states.	
She married <name> on <date>, her childhood sweetheart whom she had known for fifteen years.	Provide brief marriage details.	
She received her undergraduate degree in biology from <name of school>, attended Harvard University Medical School, and completed her residency at <name of hospital>.	Education details	
Dr. Swanson managed a privately owned clinic in Montreal for twenty-five years before retiring in <year>.	Employment details	
Preceding her in death were <names>.	List immediate family that passed away before her. Okay to list grandparents, aunts, and uncles if space permits.	

(continued)

Table 14.3. (*continued*)

Sample Phrases	Details to Collect	Notes
She is survived by <names>.	List grandparents, parents, children, sisters- and brothers-in-law, and number of great grandchildren. Edit later if you need to narrow for space.	
Dr. Swanson's heart was devoted to the community, many of whom she delivered during her thirty-five years as a family physician in her town.	Statements about your loved one's life. Include charitable work and donations.	
She was an avid golfer and five-time winner of the Montreal Golf Classic.	Highlight achievements in education, hobbies, parenting, and so on.	
The family will receive friends and loved ones at <name of funeral home and address> from <inclusive times> on <date>. Memorial services celebrating her life will be held at <location> on <date, time>. Graveside ceremony will be at <name of cemetery>.	Date, time, place of visitation, and funeral	
Rabbi Jonas Barnhart will officiate at her funeral service.	List officiate, pallbearers, and honorary pallbearers.	
The family requests that donations be sent to <name of charity>, address and <attention to>.	Do you wish donations to be sent? Will they be earmarked?	
You swept our hearts and showed us how to love.	Close with an upbeat message.	

Ask someone to proofread the obituary for the following:

- Correct spelling of deceased person's name (Many life insurance companies comb obituaries to confirm the death of beneficiaries.)

- Any names of surviving family members you may have missed

- Remove any reference to your address (City and state are enough.)

When Family Members Don't Agree

Have you ever heard these phrases?

- "I don't care what's in the will—that's not the way it's going to happen!"

- "Why did he put you in charge?"

- "I cannot stand that preacher. He'd better not say one word to me about the way I live."

Death may bring relief to the patient, but family and friends are unlikely to be as prepared for death as the caregiver. Death comes when the individual is ready, not when friends and family are ready. Count on outbursts, unusual behavior, or seemingly unkind comments that often demonstrate the person's difficulty processing death. People often are embarrassed at their behavior after the funeral. Decide in advance to let unkind comments roll off you. You have been preparing for this moment in your mind and heart, but it's pretty unlikely that friends and family are as emotionally prepared as you. In chapter 10, we provided communications guidance to help the family through financial and emotional distress as your loved one's medical crises started piling up.

Bereavement counselors agree that family members will attempt a show of strength, but inside they are paddling through grief, loneliness, anxiety, fatigue, spirituality, and mortality, among other emotions they may not be able to name. Expect flare-ups from a family member who did not take time or was unable to resolve differences with the deceased.

Some of the rules in Sabrina Alexis's article "7 Rules for Dealing with Difficult People" offer some quick tips to help you through issue resolution:

1. *The president rule:* Invite a clergy or someone who is held in high esteem to meet with all family members. Clergy are trained to listen without reproach but also to confirm your role as caregiver and executor trustee. Select someone the family respects, as this person's voice will serve as a quiet endorsement of you and the job you have ahead of you.

2. *The twenty-four-hour rule:* Listen and jot down a few notes of the concern. Then explain that the issue requires more time than you have right now to address. "How about if we talk this through after the funeral?" If the person persists, repeat your promise to revisit the issue after the funeral.

3. *The elephant rule:* If you saw an elephant storming toward you, you would step aside. When you see someone with bitterness coming your way, don't provoke or try to argue. He or she will always have an answer. Lean on

the twenty-four-hour rule after the bitter person has had some sleep and nourishment.

4. *The madhouse rule:* If you hear someone inside a "madhouse" yelling at you, you would think, "Poor guy, he's in the madhouse, but he thinks he's in charge." Everyone has issues, so put crazy requests in perspective. You don't have to comply with the loudest person in the room, but ask yourself if you would consider the request if it came from someone you respected.

Cool Tools

- *Federal Trade Commission:* Provides guidance on funerals, including how to obtain death certificates and permissions you will need to sign, such as to transport a body or to bury, embalm, or cremate the body.

- *Funeral etiquette:* Emily Post provides guidance on what to wear, when to arrive, and how to participate in processionals and recessionals. We also found an excellent guide to funeral etiquette from the Freitag Funeral Home in New Jersey.

- *Sample funeral programs:* Count on Pinterest to provide a selection of styles, language, and photos. Take these designs and customize them for your family. Print them at nearby print shops or ask the funeral director for competitive print costs.

- *Eulogies:* Sample eulogies are available at multiple websites. We found a collection of eulogies at Write-Out-Loud.com, Funeral helper.org, and Inspirationaleulogy.com.

- *Federal Trade Commission Worksheet for Funeral Costs Planning:* This site provides detailed guidance on topics many may feel too squeamish to raise. As the FTC regulates funeral services, this is a good site to learn what's allowed and what is not.

I.   "Simple" disposition of the remains:
     Immediate burial _____
     Immediate cremation _____
II. If the cremation process is extra, how much is it? _____
III. Donation of the body to a medical school or hospital _____
IV. "Traditional," full-service burial or cremation _____
V.   Basic services fee for the funeral director and staff _____
     Pickup of body _____
     Embalming _____

Other preparation of body _____

Least expensive casket _____

Description, including model number _____

Outer burial container (vault) _____

Description _____

VI. Visitation/viewing—staff and facilities _____

Funeral or memorial service—staff and facilities _____

Graveside service, including staff and equipment _____

VII. Hearse _____

Other vehicles _____

Total _____

VIII. Other services:

Forwarding body to another funeral home _____

Receiving body from another funeral home _____

IX. Cemetery/mausoleum costs:

Cost of lot or crypt (if you don't already own one) _____

Perpetual care _____

Opening and closing the grave or crypt _____

Grave liner, if required _____

Marker/monument (including setup) _____

Section 3 has dealt with some pretty tough issues, all of them part of being the caregiver. Chapter 16 focuses on you and your healing. We provide guidance on how to reclaim yourself—the person you were before you took on caregiving responsibilities compared to the person you want to be now.

Key Takeaways

In this chapter, you learned the following:

- Funerals are events that require preplanning. No one will evaluate whether it was well done, but everyone will admire you if you allow them to help. Give them a task, then step out of the way and let them help. It won't be done the way you would have done it, but it will be done with love.

- How to build a budget and stick with the plan. Ask a businessperson whom you admire to be your advocate when fulfilling your loved one's funeral wishes.

- Consider yourself among the lucky ones if your loved one purchased funeral arrangements prior to passing. Prepaid funeral plans may become complex if your loved one purchased a plan in one state and then moved to another to live with family.

■ Surround yourself with people who help you stay centered. Emotional reactions to things you hear and say are a normal part of the funeral. Let go as quickly as you can of comments that were said in the heat of the moment.

15 Closing Out Accounts

This chapter begins with an explanation of notifications that should automatically be put in place when an individual is declared deceased, such as notifications to the Social Security Administration and what happens to bank accounts, credit card accounts, and insurance accounts. We provide guidance on how to consolidate funds, wills, trusts, and the probate process when there is a will.

We also provide guidance on the following:

- Tasks the funeral company should do and what they might do to help close accounts.

- The difference between having power of attorney and the executor trustee, including the responsibilities and authority granted to you from your loved one's will.

- Sample letters to send to credit card agencies, insurance policies, and other participants in the loved one's financial portfolio.

This chapter is loaded with checklists that are provided in the book and also downloaded from Caregivers-Toolbox.com In this chapter, you also will find sample letters to send when closing out accounts, spreadsheets to track responses, and how credit reports are an important part of preventive theft as well as closing accounts.

After the Funeral

The funeral or memorial service is over, and friends and relatives have gone. Whether it has been a lengthy journey with your loved one or a sudden, unexpected life-ending event, you are more than likely exhausted, both physically and emotionally, as you grieve your loss.

What next? There are still many tasks that need to be done after the death of your loved one. One of the tasks you will need to tackle is closing out accounts.

Where do you begin? If you are the spouse or executor of the deceased person. you should immediately request certified copies of the death certificate, the official record of the date and location of your loved one's death. These can be obtained from your funeral director or requested from your city clerk's office or office of vital records. Certified copies will have a raised seal and are used for legal purposes, such as closing out financial accounts. You will need anywhere from ten to twenty copies since each account you are closing will probably require a copy of this valuable and original document.

As soon as possible after receiving the death certificate copies, you will want to begin contacting each account you wish to close. Before you can do this, though, you must gather records and documents for each account. Table 15.1 represents important documents to collect but is not all-inclusive. Take this with you to the funeral director to track what you must do and what the funeral home will do.

Table 15.1.   Documents to Be Collected

What to Collect	Status of Collection
• Death certificate(s) The funeral home can order these for you. Obtain ten to twenty copies for an adult; for a child, five to ten are adequate. You can order additional copies online at Vital Records: Vitalrec.com.	
• The will or trust Discuss or consult with your attorney on the specifics with your situation.	
• Last credit card statements Check also to see if the deceased had a life insurance policy on any credit cards.	
• Last checking statement • Last mortgage statement • Last savings account statement Validate the names on each account.	
Investment accounts • 401k • Individual retirement account • Mutual funds • Pensions • CDs • Money market accounts Validate the names on each account.	

What to Collect	Status of Collection
• Social Security card of deceased	

• Credit report of the deceased
  This can be ordered at no charge at annualcreditreport.com.
  You will need the Social Security number of the deceased.	

Last two years' income tax returns • State • Federal • W2	
• Marriage and birth certificates (of the deceased's spouse and children) • Divorce papers, if applicable	
• Automobile title and registration	
Insurance policies • Life • Umbrella • Auto • Disability • Supplement	
• Deeds and property titles	
• Car loans, student loans, etc.	

While collecting your loved one's documents, you should also begin the important process of reaching out to his or her work and support resources. Be certain to record a history of your communications with each person you contact (see table 15.2).

When a close friend died unexpectedly, we were all stunned and tried to assist his wife, who was herself recovering from a recent major medical situation. Some of her immediate concerns were "Will I still have health coverage?," "Who do I contact to let his employer know of his death?," and "Did he have life insurance?" During this time of mourning, we sat on her front porch, reminisced, and compassionately discussed whom she needed to contact to answer these questions.

(Peter Wong)

Table 15.2. People or Organizations to Contact When Closing an Account

Whom to Contact	Date Completed
Contact Health Insurance of Employer.	
Terminate coverage of the deceased while ensuring coverage for others in the family if appropriate.	
Obtain Letters of Testamentary or Letters of Administration.	
"A Letter of Testamentary—sometimes called a 'Letter of Administration' or 'Letter of Representation'—is a document granted by a local court. The document simply states that you are the legal executor for a particular estate and that you have the ability to act as such. This letter along with the death certificate are the two documents you'll need to do the real estate transactions, banking, and asset distribution you were appointed to do." (rocketlawyer.com).	
Consult an Attorney and Accountant.	
Even if you decide not to use one. The attorney and accountant should specialize in wills, trusts, and estates exclusively.	
Contact the Employer of Your Loved One.	
To determine if there are any credit union or union death benefits, the employer's human resources department can help. You will need a certified copy of the death certificate for each claim.	
Cancel or Transfer Accounts, Subscriptions and Memberships.	
These can be found by reviewing bank statements, mail, and e-mail. Examples of accounts to transfer are joint bank accounts, stocks, bonds, utility bills, and mortgage accounts. Subscriptions could include investment newsletters, magazines, etc. Membership could include auto clubs, travel groups, and airline or hotel reward programs.	
Contact Insurance Company.	
If your loved one had life insurance policies, you will need the policy number and a certified copy of the death certificate.	
If your loved one is listed as the beneficiary on any other policy, this is the appropriate time to have his or her name removed.	
Social Security Administration	
Many times, the funeral director will report it once you furnish the Social Security number of the deceased to him or her. Any benefits your loved one was receiving must be returned to Social Security for	

Whom to Contact	Date Completed
the month of death and any later months. You do not want to cash any Social Security checks received after your loved one's death because repayment is a difficult process. To make certain the family receives all benefits to which they are entitled, you may contact social security.gov.	
U.S. Military/Veterans Benefits	
The Veterans Administration may be contacted at (800) 335-2031 to determine benefits eligibility. A copy of your loved one's discharge papers will be needed and can be requested from the War Records Office located in each state.	

Veterans should also contact The Dignity Memorial Network. This is North America's largest provider of funeral, cremation, and cemetery services. Lists of additional facts regarding Veterans Administration benefits are given in table 15.3.

What Happens to Bank Accounts?

FAQ: Who becomes the owner of someone's property when he or she dies, for example, a bank account?

Table 15.3.   Veterans Death Benefits

• U.S. Department of Veterans Affairs benefits do not cover all of the funeral or cremation arrangements of honorably discharged veterans.
• You will need documentation to verify military service. A copy or verification of loved one's military discharge is needed. This can be found from the state War Records Office.
• A "Presidential Memorial Certificate" must be requested.
• Veterans buried in a private cemetery may be eligible for partial reimbursement. In order to determine any reimbursement amount, the family must complete an Application for Burial Benefits (VA Form 21-530).
• Request for issuance of replacement medals or awards must be requested in writing. The request should be made to the National Personnel Records Center (NPRC) at (866) 272-6272 or by visiting the NPRC website at Archive.gov.
• Headstones or military markers are available from the Veterans Administration on request. • An Application for Standard Government Headstone or Marker (VA Form 40-1330) is required.

Answer: Sometimes understanding what happens to bank accounts is easy. In a joint account that the deceased owned with a loved one, on death the loved one becomes the sole owner of the account. The account will not go through probate court for approval.

Example: Alice and Lenny have a bank account together, a joint account. The statement reads "Alice OR Lenny." On Lenny's death, Alice becomes the sole owner of the account and can close the account if she wishes.

Other scenarios can require more understanding, such as a bank account with a payable-on-death (POD) beneficiary The bank may also call this a custodial account, a transfer on death account, or a totem trust account. The deceased has made the transfer of the account to one or more persons easy by filling out a form designating the account's POD beneficiary. Once the person dies, the money in the account is quickly transferred to the POD beneficiary, and the account will not have to go through probate court for approval.

Example: Lenny owns a bank account in his name alone and has named Alice as the POD beneficiary. On Lenny's death, Alice will provide the bank with a certified death certificate, and the money in the account will be given to her.

A slightly more complex scenario of transferring assets at death is a bank account created as a trust account. This gives a safe haven for assets as they are being passed on or used on behalf of the account beneficiaries.

Example: Lenny created a trust account, meaning that the bank account he opened is owned by his trust. The statement reads, "The Lenny Revocable Trust." Lenny is the trustee of the account and can access the account during his life. The trust states that Alice will automatically become the trustee when Lenny dies, at which time she must close the account and give the money to Debbie. When Lenny dies, Alice will provide the bank with a certified copy of the death certificate and the trust provision naming her as the new trustee. The bank will close the account and give the money to Alice. Alice will then follow the instructions of the trust account and give the money to Debbie.

FAQ: What happens when power of attorney(POA) is involved in a bank account?

Answer: The POA's access ends when the loved one dies unless the POA's name also is listed on the account.

Example: Lenny has a bank account in his name alone but has given Alice the power of attorney to access the account in order to pay his bills if he becomes sick or otherwise incapacitated. The statement reads, "Lenny. Alice, POA (Power of Attorney)" The right given to Alice to access this account ends on Lenny's death. No one can access the account after Lenny's death without the permission of a probate court judge.

Our final example is Lenny having a bank account in his name alone. No one else has the right to access the account, and no one can access the account after Lenny's death without the permission of a probate court judge.

FAQ: What is probate?

Answer: Probate is establishing the validity of a will in a court of law. The probate process is time consuming, allows public knowledge of your assets, and can be expensive. It is not uncommon for a deceased person's account to be in probate up to two years.

FAQ: How can you avoid probate?

Answer: Many people try to avoid family members having to wade through probate after their death by establishing the following:

- Joint ownership on all financial and real estate accounts.

- Revocable or living trusts.

- Beneficiary named on all assets. It is important to have a beneficiary on all financial, insurance, and investment accounts.

- Do not name your estate (property or possession) as beneficiary.

What Happens to Credit Cards?

In chapter 4, we showed you how to request a free copy of your loved one's credit report at Annualcreditreport.com. After the death of your loved one, you can use the report to identify open credit card accounts and begin to close them. Until the estate is settled, it is a good idea to check the credit reports every six months to ensure that no fraudulent accounts have been opened in the deceased's name.

When closing credit cards for your loved one, remember that power of attorney ends at death. You do not have authority to cancel your loved one's credit cards after death unless you are the executor of the will or you are the administrator of the estate without a will.

To begin the account closing process, you will need to send a letter to the credit card company with the following information: (1) the account name, (2) the account number, (3) a certified copy of the death certificate, and (4) a postage-paid return envelope. It is important to keep a record of confirmation that the account has been closed.

You may be asked to settle any amount owed to the credit card company. If it was a joint credit card account, any remaining balance owed may be passed on to the person named on the account. Some credit card companies have forgiven debts owed to them on death, while others have asked the estate to settle the balance. It is recommended that you have a discussion with the credit card company, as they resolve on a case-to-case basis.

What Happens to Insurance Accounts?

In order to receive money from a life insurance policy owned by your deceased loved one, you must be the beneficiary, file a claim, and provide the policy number and a certified death certificate. You may also be asked to provide a W-9 form to the Internal Revenue Service if any interest on the policy was paid to you. It is important to document your conversations with the insurance company.

There may often be additional benefits owed to the beneficiary because of other life insurance policies the deceased took out without informing the beneficiary. It is up to the beneficiary to locate these, as insurance companies may not be attempting to track you down. The author has personally experienced this while helping friends locate policies several years after the death of their loved ones.

At times, insurance companies turn death benefits over as unclaimed property when they know that the policyholder is deceased. So if you don't know the name of your loved one's insurance company, you may want to begin your search with the National Association of Unclaimed Property Administrators at NAUPA.

There are many types of insurance accounts. We recommend that you check to see if your loved one purchased any of these:

- *Individual insurance policy:* The policy could be located in the safe-deposit box.

- *Group insurance policy:* Usually obtained through employer, professional or social organization, bank, or credit agency.

- *Employee-based insurance policy:* Check with the employer. Also look at pay stubs that may document your loved one's payments. Discuss with the human resources and benefits departments of your loved one's employer.

- *Credit life insurance:* Banks and lenders provide credit life insurance through loans or lines of credit to individuals. The credit insurance is often bundled with the individual's loan or credit line. This insurance pays off the loan in the event of the individual's death. Check with banks and lenders to see if a policy was purchased by your loved one.

- *Mortgage life insurance:* Life insurance policies are incorporated into the mortgage payments and will pay off the mortgage on death. Check with the mortgage lender on this benefit.

- *Accidental death policy:* Check with the employer, as many employees sign up for this additional benefit. A secondary source for accidental death benefits consists of credit card policies or airline travel policies. Check credit card terms and conditions as well as individual travel ticket invoices. Car rental and travel services also provide accidental death policies.

Sample Letters

Here we provide sample letters for you to customize when reaching out to financial institutions. Before submitting the letter, be sure you provide what they seek, which likely includes the following:

- Death certificate with raised seal.

- Pages from the trust document naming you executor of the estate, including any notarized or witnesses pages.

- Women who remarried and changed their name after being named the executrix must also provide a marriage certificate explaining any name changes.

- Deceased's policy number.

Power of Attorney

The power of attorney is a legal document that gives a person you choose (your agent) the authority to manage your affairs while you are living. The power of attorney allows your agent to manage your finances, legal matters, and health care decisions, among other things. The power of attorney ends when your loved one dies.

A common misconception about power of attorney is thinking that the agent will continue to have legal authority after the loved one's death and will be able to settle the estate and close accounts. Remember, the power of attorney and its authority end when your loved one dies. If the power of attorney also is named the executor trustee in the will, then that role transitions to manage the estate.

Figure 15.1. Sample Letter to a Financial Institution

[Your name]
[Address line 1]
[Address line 2]

[Financial Institution]
[Address line 1]
[Address line 2]

[Date]

To whom it may concern (Name appropriate)

Re [name of deceased]
Investment(s): [Account numbers(s)]

I am the personal representative of [deceased] who died on [date]. Enclosed is a certified copy of the death certificate, which I would like returned to me once you have noted the details. I am enclosing a postage-paid envelope for your convenience.

Please advise me of any survivor value now payable and of any other benefits for the deceased's beneficiaries. I would also like to close the account effective [date].

Please let me know how to proceed and what further information you need.

I can be reached by email at xxxx@xxxx.com or by phone at xxx-xxx-1234.

Kind Regards,

[Your signature]

[Your name]

NOTE: You may also be required to provide pages from the deceased's trust document to verify that you are the executor.

Figure 15.2.   Sample Letter for a Membership or Subscription:

[Your name]
[Address line 1]
[Address line 2]

[Membership or Subscription]
[Address line 1]
[Address line 2]

[Date]

To whom it may concern (Name appropriate)

Re [name of deceased]
Membership(s): [Account numbers(s)]

I am the personal representative of [deceased] who died on [date]. Enclosed is a certified copy of the death certificate, which I would like returned to me once you have noted the details. I am enclosing a postage-paid envelope for your convenience.

Please advise me of any survivor value now payable and of any other benefits for the deceased's beneficiaries. I would also like to transfer the membership/subscription to [Your name].

Please let me know how to proceed and what further information you need.

I can be reached by email at xxxx@xxxx.com or by phone at xxx-xxx-1234.

Kind Regards,

[Your signature]

[Your name]

Figure 15.3. Sample Letter for an Insurance Policy

[Your name]
[Address line 1]
[Address line 2]

[Insurance Company]
[Address line 1]
[Address line 2]

[Date]

To whom it may concern (Name appropriate)

Re [name of deceased]
Policy number(s): [Claim numbers(s)]

I am the personal representative of [deceased] who died on [date]. Enclosed is a certified copy of the death certificate, which I would like returned to me once you have noted the details. I am enclosing a postage-paid envelope for your convenience.

Please advise me of the value of the deceased's life insurance policy, any survivor value now payable, and any other benefits for the deceased's beneficiaries.

Please let me know how to proceed and what further information you need.

I can be reached by email at xxxx@xxxx.com or by phone at xxx-xxx-1234.

Kind Regards,

[Your signature]

[Your name]

Figure 15.4. Sample Letter to Close a Credit Card Account

[Your name]
[Address line 1]
[Address line 2]

[Credit Card Company]
[Address line 1]
[Address line 2]

[Date]

To whom it may concern (Name appropriate)

Re [name of deceased]
Credit Card(s): [Account Number(s)]

I am writing to close the above credit card account.

I am the personal representative of [deceased] who died on [date]. Enclosed is a certified copy of the death certificate, which I would like returned to me once you have noted the details. I have enclosed a postage-paid envelope for your convenience.

Please acknowledge closure of this account in writing.

I can be reached by email at xxxx@xxxx.com or by phone at xxx-xxx-1234 if there are any questions.

Kind Regards,

[Your signature]

[Your name]

Table 15.4. Sample Spreadsheet to Track Letter Responses

Using a spreadsheet is helpful in tracking the responses you receive from the organizations you have contacted regarding closing an account. This list can be expanded and customized for your personal use. Create your own blank form or download a blank spreadsheet at Caregivers-Toolbox.com.

Organization	Date Sent	Response	Follow-Up Date	Completed Date	Death Certificate Sent
American Express	October 12	Yes	October 15		Yes
Chase Bank/Visa	October 12		October 15		Yes
Attorney	October 12	Yes	October 13		Yes
Accountant					Yes
Employer	October 10	Yes			Yes
401k, Merrill Lynch	October 14	Yes			Yes
Individual retirement account, Vanguard	October 14				Yes
Social Security	October 10	Yes			Yes
Veterans Affairs	October 10				Yes
New York Life Insurance	October 10	Yes			Yes

Cool Tools

- *Power of attorney forms for each state:* Includes multiple types of power of attorney forms, including durable, general, limited, and medical, for each state.

- The following websites offer power of attorney forms for free, but you may be charged a fee for some purchases you make on these sites:

  - TotalLegal.com

  - LawDepot.com

  - RocketLawyer.com

Executor

The executor is a person named by the deceased in his or her will to direct the distribution of the deceased's estate. The loved one chose this person while still living. A probate court of law will establish the validity of the loves one's will and appoint the executor as named. If your loved one died without a will, the probate court will appoint a person called an administrator to distribute the estate of the deceased. The role of the executor includes gathering assets, collecting debts, paying bills, and closing accounts.

Cool Tools

- *Executor roles and duties:* FindLaw.com provides roles and duties of the executor.

Key Takeaways

In this chapter, you learned the following:

- Fifteen or more notarized copies of the death certificate should be obtained, as each account to be closed will likely require an original certificate.

- Key pages within the will that state that you are the executor trustee should be made. Keep a scanned copy in your electronic file, as you will need to access this many times. Key pages include front and back pages that include signatures, witnesses and notary, and paragraphs that identify you as executor trustee.

- Women identified as executor trustee under their maiden name but have since married must provide a copy of the marriage certificate to each account.

- The executor trustee named in the will should close accounts owned by the deceased.

16 | Reclaim Yourself

Caregiving does a number on you, to your heart, to your personal and professional life, and to your inherent value system. You don't have to wait until your role as caregiver stops to reclaim yourself. Ideally, this is an ongoing process. But when you stop providing care for whatever reason, you will need time to heal, reidentify, and reeducate yourself.

The world changed while you were caring for a loved one, making it tough to find work or reapply your skills in a current work environment. You also changed. You may have been part of the $570+ billion unpaid "informal" care partners, but now you need to turn that into a productive, paying job.

Michael T. S. Lindenmayer, founder of the Caregiver Relief Fund, says, "We need a nationwide caregiver makeover session. Plan or Perish."

In this chapter, we provide advice from others who have walked where you are to find guidance on the following:

- Acknowledging your feelings.

- Using what you learned as a caregiver to help others.

- Going back to work.

- Reestablishing relationships.

Acknowledging Your Feelings

You are who you were before giving care but now you are so much wiser and softer. You had to be strong for the person you cared for, and now the reason for that strength is gone. Your faith was likely a refuge for you, a place where you could share frustrations and express mixed emotions about your loved one's response to you.

After caregiving, caregivers often feel profound fatigue, guilt, or anger with the medical processes that should not have happened or that should have but didn't. A friend of ours said the best way to get over depression is to get into it. Feel it, acknowledge it, but don't bypass it because it will lurk in the shadows, masking itself until it comes out as a life-threatening disease.

Spend a day deep in tears. Stay hydrated but cry it out. Write it out, shout it out, but get it out. Some may need professional guidance through complicated grief.

Talk about the death and the life of your loved one if it helps. This may also be an opportunity for your support group to share their feelings with you.

Count on the passage of time to make things better, but there is no normal time period for grief. People grieve in stages.

I went back to my mom's home alone a month after she passed away so that I could determine what to do with her personal items. Other family members would arrive soon, but I wanted first to be alone with her things, smelling her and feeling her spirit in the home. In going through her jewelry, her clothes, and secret notes she filed in her Bible, I felt like I was violating her most private world as I tried to determine what to keep, what to share with friends and family, and what to throw away. Old paint cans and empty jars were easy to pitch. It was in the scrapbooks she had kept since childhood that I learned about the days she sang and served as a waitress on the Great Lakes cruises in the 1940s. I read about her saddest times as a mom when my sister's fever spiked to 106 and about the joy she felt in giving birth to my brother. As I slept in her empty bed, I listened to a CD that Michael Taylor, my friend and beloved church pianist in Swansboro, North Carolina, had recorded, "Great Hymns of the Heart." I let myself lean into my sadness and felt her joy in being with my father, my brother, and my sister in Heaven. I let the music soothe me to whatever sleep I would be allowed that night, knowing that I needed to go deeply into depression after caring for her for so many years. It was that night of acknowledging my deep sadness that allowed me to finally get up the next morning and begin closing out her home, a place of joy and laughter, a kitchen where so many people from the Gallatin Baptist Church gathered for dinner and her over-sweetened apple pies. That next day, I sat at her organ and piano and tapped out the songs she loved so much. I found her old scratchy choir recordings and played them as I reopened her will, making sure that her treasures made it into piles marked for each grandchild. As family members arrived to help, I was able to guide them through their grief, welcoming a place now and then to stop and share tears, laughter, and a great glass of wine.

(Carolyn Hartley)

Reclaim Yourself Even If the Disease Is in Remission

If your loved one recovered and returned to live a modified but full life, you still must find your place again in the relationship. Your loved one may not want to be cared for any more. "You have to let me do this myself," he might say.

The American Society of Clinical Oncology's Cancer.net provides helpful guidance on what to do if your loved one no longer needs your help.

1. *Acknowledge that the disease is in remission:* "The two scariest days in a cancer patient's life are the day they were diagnosed and the day they are released from treatment," said Patricia Ganz, MD, a pioneer in advocating for patients and their families, earning her a place among Best Doctors in America. "Remission," she said, "is the beginning of a five-year clock. Everyone holds their breath but you have to get on with your life."

2. *Understand the disease:* Young adults in particular need help coping after cancer. Give yourself time to adjust to physical and emotional changes.

3. *Connect with others who have achieved remission:* As a caregiver, you would recognize the back story behind six-time all-star pitcher Curt Schilling, now an ESPN analyst, who also knows what it's like to be a caregiver for his wife, Shonda, also in remission. Perhaps you publicly watched the battle of Dr. Jen Arnold, star of *The Little Couple*, or Robin Roberts, cohost of *Good Morning America*, and her grateful attribution to family and her girlfriend, Amber.

4. *Resume activities:* Continue doing things you enjoy or dedicate time to a new hobby.

5. *Take care of your body:* Stay hydrated and get back into a regular sleep pattern. No one knows more than new parents and caregivers how sleep deprivation can affect your health.

6. *Connect with a community:* Join a new book club, create a supper club, or get back in touch with friends whose company you enjoy.

7. *Become a cancer advocate:* People who have survived cancer offer positive and encouraging support to those living with cancer. Write in a journal. Your private thoughts help relieve some of the stresses and can be a powerful antidote for you and your personal pain.

Using What You Learned as a Caregiver

Caregivers develop skills they never thought they would need. During the period you were a caregiver, you learned how to fulfill the following roles:

Researcher
Project manager

Stress manager

Wellness manager

Problem solver

Negotiator

Financial officer

Time manager

Writer

And much more!

Learn more about how your skills help position you for a career. We suggest that you participate in a skills assessment, offered either at your local community college or online at career placement centers.

Cool Tools for Assessing Your Skills

- *ISEEK Careers:* This allows you to create a free account and then complete an assessment. Using results of your assessment, you can search for specific careers that match your profile.

- *Monster.com:* One of the largest online job search engines, this also provides skills assessment guidance. In an article by Carole Martin, she recalls how one woman packaged herself with a list of ingredients or skills she had to offer. Using three P's, she categorized herself into the following:

  1. Previous experience

     - Some of the entries offered here included marketing knowledge, communication skills, Web channel marketing, and computer skills.

  2. Portable skills

     - Portable skills referred to skills that transition from one employer to another, such as customer focused, writing skills, and team leader.

  3. Personality traits

     - Personality attributions included self-starter, independent, problem solver, good judgment, analytical, and good sense of humor.

Going Back to Work

In a study of daughters who cared for an elderly parent managing Alzheimer's or a related disease, researchers found two great reasons to hire caregivers over noncaregivers:

1. Caregivers had a better sense of well-being and ability to manage stress. Their skills as caregivers equipped them with skills to "mobilize and utilize resources and support systems and develop a management approach" to problem solving.

2. Caregivers had a better life balance and more maturity and focused on strengths-based interventions aimed at operations. Caregivers could quickly reprioritize realistic goals and identify formal and informal needs.

This study, "Comparing the Well-Being of Post-Caregivers and Non-Caregivers," funded by the Alzheimer's Disease and Related Disorders Program at the University of Missouri, Columbia, also found that postcaregivers earned higher wages than noncaregivers.

Work is what you need it to be to feel productive. Going back to work may mean hiring a contractor to remodel the bedroom or kitchen. Work may also mean taking up a new hobby or taking what you have learned and turning it into a business. Seek counsel from a college career center that offers business management advice at reduced hourly costs or join the chamber of commerce and learn what's available in your region.

Deborah Shouse, author of *Love in the Land of Dementia: Finding Hope in the Caregiver's Journey*, writes about how to celebrate and appreciate what we have right now. Shouse says that she discovered compassion, deepening love, and increased connection with her mother and family during the time her mother transitioned through dementia, memory loss, and Alzheimer's disease. In working with her life partner, she and Ron Zoglin perform her stories to live audiences, raising more than $80,000 for Alzheimer's programs and research.

Reestablishing Relationships

Women often say they find the "renewed me" in yoga, craft classes, book clubs, or volunteering for a caregiving organization to give back the support they had received. Some go after a job promotion that may have evaded them during the caregiving years. Others register at community colleges to learn a trade that emerged while they were caregiving. Men often join breakfast clubs, join fitness clubs, or return to a Sunday school class.

Start or participate in a blog. RightatHome.net recommends several blogs for caregivers. We liked some of those that provided a forum for anyone to post a comment. As each blog has its own personality and author requirements, check out each before you post:

- *Alzheimer's Reading Room:* The blog focuses primarily on readers' responses to articles that have been syndicated in other news sources.

- *The Caregiver's Voice:* This blog gives advice and encouragement.

- *Caring.com Blogs:* This blog is a well-read website that offers advice from experts on family tensions, geriatrics, self-care, and technology.

- *eCare Diary:* The focus here is on simplifying the life of a caregiver.

- *Eldercare ABC (About Being Connected):* This blog promises to establish a community of bloggers who care for both their children and their aging parents.

Put down the technology, walk across the street, and reintroduce yourself to your neighbors. They already know why you've been put out of commission. If you aren't sure what to say, try any of these conversation starters:

- "Hi, my name is <Carolyn Hartley>. I've been fairly preoccupied for a while and thought I'd reintroduce myself." (This usually gets a grin, especially if you say you are Carolyn Hartley or Peter Wong.)

- "I've been staying up pretty late. Any recommendations on late-night snacks?"

- "I noticed your grandkids have been here this summer. How are they doing?"

- "Who do you recommend for house painting? I'm planning to redo my office."

Cool Tools

- *Return to handcrafts:* Reclaim Yourself Retreat brings women together to make gifts and holiday decor; enjoy delicious meals and desserts; learn new techniques for scrapbooking, needle crafting, quilting, and painting; or advertise products you are making. Nothing has to be perfect. You're on the rebound.

- *Take a cruise:* Royal Caribbean Cruise Lines features a Caregiver Spa Getaway. Take care of yourself and make new friends with other veteran caregivers. Share new problem-solving techniques while people pamper you.

- *Join a class:* Join a yoga, supper club, exercise, writing, or Sunday school class.

- *Take a class at a community college:* The cost of these classes typically ranges from $15 to $75 per session; no one cares if you pass or fail.

- *Learn something new:* Learn how to sail. Learn how to paint. Buy a sheet of lumber and ask the sales rep to cut it into sections for you.

- *Meditate:* Invite the presence of positive energy to strengthen you.

- *Energize your senses:* Listen to music. Read a book. Taste new foods or drinks. Try your hand at pottery.

- *Get certified in your professional field:* Getting certified often means increased salary. Jobs that require you have certification tend to pay more than jobs that don't. Go to HowToGetCertified.com. At this site, you can select the school or program that is right for you.

- *Start or join a caregiver's blog:* You may want to teach something, make people laugh or tell your story in short segments. Wikihow.com/Start-a-Blog offers terrific advice on how to start a blog, what to write, and how to get people to read your blog or even post a link from their log to yours.

- *Volunteer:* Your hard-won skills are someone else's coaching. Volunteer at a senior center, hospital, church, or synagogue.

Key Takeaways

In this chapter, you learned the following:

- How to acknowledge your feelings, your joys, and your sorrows so that you can create a new productive life for yourself.

- How to leverage what you learned as a caregiver to help others. Employers often find that caregivers are those who can multitask, caregivers anticipate and plan rather than jump in and react, and caregivers are some of the first to step up and take on new responsibilities.

- Going back to full-time work requires support from friends and colleagues. You may also need to manage your workload at first.

- Reestablish relationships with friends who you weren't always able to connect with while you were caring for a loved one.

- You are on a new path. Surround yourself with joy and love by sharing your story with others who can learn from you.

Epilogue

We listened to dozens of caregivers while writing this book, and we learned so many things about the heart of caregivers, care partners, and their loved ones along the way.

Carolyn learned that in hiring fourteen employees and subcontractors for her company, Physicians EHR, that all of them turned out to be caregivers, taking care of a loved one for less than one year or many years. She did not intend to hire caregivers for her health technology and patient engagement company. However, the inherent qualities required to service high-stakes, high-risk physician practices was a great match with professionals who also understood the technical, legal, and compliance restrictions physicians have when communicating with patients and family. Carolyn also learned that her caregiving employees could best meet their work performance goals when she brought the process of caregiving away from watercooler gossip and into the mainstream. Many of the mobile apps provided in this book also were tested by our friends, families, and workforce. Moved by the incredible spirit of caregivers, Carolyn has devoted much of her professional work to help physicians and hospital staff meet quality improvement measures that engage patients in the healing process.

Peter's heart has long been devoted to supporting caregivers, especially through his work with faith communities. At one time, he believes he was guarded about sharing caregiving stories with the chief executive officers (CEOs), board chairs, or high-level executives for which he provided strategic risk management guidance. But when he began talking with CEO-level friends about the book he was writing, he learned that many were eager to share their stories. Many were at the crossroads of caring for parents while leading an executive team. Peter listened to their vulnerability and prayed with them for strength, wisdom, and courage. He also saw an increase in questions employers started asking about wellness programs that would help offset the cost of health care benefits, improve productivity, and reduce the increasing divide between benefits and salaries. His approach to risk management also helped health care professionals take another look at the care they were providing to patients and the potential to miss important communication with caregivers.

To that end, we hope to actively observe and educate employers as the trend to assist caregiver employees becomes part of the mainstream workplace.

Tell us what you need or tell us about tools in this book that have helped you. Take time to post your story at Caregivers-Toolbox.com. Or e-mail us at Carolyn.Hartley@caregivers-toolbox.com or Peter.Wong@caregivers-Toolbox.com.

Glossary

Terms in *the Caregiver's Toolbox* are provided for educational value and simplified for understandability. They are not intended to be used for any legal decisions but are for the benefit of our readers.

Access: In HIPAA, this refers to the availability of medical care and permissions given to certain users to access protected health information. Some people in rural or underserved areas have a difficult time accessing medical care. *See also* Telemedicine.

Accidental Death Policy: An insurance policy typically issued through the employer or credit card company. Insurance coverage is in the event of death due to travel-related activities, such as an accident.

Accountant: A person who audits and keeps the financial records of an individual.

Accounting of Disclosures: This is a request you make with your health care professional asking for a list of people and organizations that received a copy of your or your loved one's medical or dental chart.

Advance Directive: Legal documents that spell out the end-of-life wishes ahead of time for yourself or your loved one.

Affordable Care Act: Federal statute effective March 2010 that is part of the health care reform agenda signed by President Obama. The law includes provisions that include the expansion of Medicaid eligibility, keeps young adults covered, ends arbitrary withdrawal of insurance coverage if you made an honest mistake, grants the right of appeal if your insurance company denies a payment, bans lifetime limits on benefits, enables health insurance exchanges, requires health plans to publicly justify rate hikes, and prohibits health insurers from denying coverage due to preexisting conditions.

Aging in Place: The ability for one to live in one's own home safely as long as he or she is able, as he or she grows older.

Amend: In HIPAA, this means you can request to alter a document that you believe is incorrect. For example, your chart says you broke your left arm when you actually broke your right arm. The health care professional who built your medical chart will approve or deny your request to amend. If you wish to change something that is medically accurate, your request will be denied.

Antivirus Software: Software that is used to prevent the infiltration of viruses to one's information technology or network.

Authorization: More specific than consent to disclose information. An authorization must be dated and is for a specific purpose. For example, your provider wants to send you an e-mail inviting you to join a patient portal. You can sign this authorization but the practice also promises to keep your confidential health information secure. No one except you and your doctor can review the contents.

Beneficiary: The person or group who receives benefits under health care insurance.

Blog: An informational site where discussions can be held over the Internet.

Breach: An unauthorized disclosure of your health information indicating that the confidentiality of your health information may have been exposed to someone who shouldn't have access to it. Providers are required by law to notify you of a breach and what they are doing to secure your protected health information. They also must provide you with credit-monitoring services for a specified amount of time. In cases where 500 or more individuals are affected, the media also must be notified of the breach.

Caregiver: In the context of this book, a caregiver is someone who cares for another person who is sick, elderly, or disabled and who does not get paid for the services.

Centers for Medicare and Medicaid Services (CMS): The federal agency within the U.S. Department of Health and Human Services that covers insurance for more than 100 million people eligible for Medicare, Medicaid, the Children's Health Insurance Program, and the Health Insurance Marketplace. CMS also supports clinical quality measures to achieve a high-quality health system at lower costs.

Certified Eldercare Law Attorney (CELA): Certification for lawyers who specialize in elder law and pass criteria and education on elder law.

Checking Statement: A statement from a financial institution that shows the check history of an account.

Claim Detail: Detailed accounting of each service provided, itemized by procedure code. Procedure codes (CPT) align with diagnosis codes (ICD), and when they don't, the payer may deny the claim. You have a much better chance of negotiating a claim if you have a detailed claim, but you also may need to consult a professional advocate to understand what the codes mean.

Clinical Summary: An after-visit summary that provides the patient with information relevant to this office visit and action items you agree to do following the appointment. Clinical summaries include the provider's contact information, date and location of visit, an updated medication list, updated vitals, and procedures completed or to be ordered. Most physicians offer a clinical summary after each visit. They also may post your summary on a patient portal.

Clinical Trial: A controlled clinical investigation to determine the outcomes and efficiency of a drug, vaccines, medical device, or surgical procedure. Clinical trials typically are regulated by the Food and Drug Administration.

Communication Plan: A plan that ensures that the family and friends of the loved one receive proper and timely information about the situation.

Confidential Communications: This describes where you want to be reached and also provides permission for health or dental professionals to leave a message on your voice mail or speak to another member of your family. For example, you wish to always be reached on your mobile phone, and you also give the provider permission to discuss protected health information with your spouse.

Consent to Disclose Information: Different from a consent to treat, this gives the health care professional permission to disclose a minimum amount of information about your care and treatment to individuals or organizations. Providers do not need your consent to share information with other providers engaged in your care, but many ask you to sign this form as a courtesy, letting you know they will submit information about you to your health plan.

Consent to Treatment: A form used by health care professionals to obtain your consent prior to performing a medical procedure or treatment. Most consumers sign consent to treat but often neglect to ask about the costs of the procedure or treatment prior to signing.

Covered Entities: Covered entity is a health care professional, a health plan, or a clearinghouse that must comply with HIPAA Privacy, Security, and Breach Notification Rules. A covered entity engages in the electronic exchange of protected health information for reimbursement.

Credit Life Insurance: A type of life insurance that is often bundled with the individual's loan or credit line. This insurance pays off the loan in the event of the individual's death.

Death Certificate: A legal document that certifies that one is deceased. It is signed by a doctor and provides the name of the deceased, sex, age, and time and cause of death.

Debit Card: Sometimes called a bank card or check card, a plastic card for payment that provides access to one's bank account at a financial institution. The card can be used instead of cash for purchases. Debit cards have more liability than do credit cards.

Deed: A legal document that has been signed, sealed, and delivered by an individual granting property to another individual.

Diagnosis: A clinical conclusion made by a health care provider following a careful examination of an individual's medical history.

Digital Legacy: A compilation of the technology you use every day to make your life run more smoothly. It may be e-mail, Facebook, e-banking, online bill payment options, or anything that deals with tracking your personal assets.

Disease Discovery: The process of analyzing data to identify the diagnosis. This comes from the patient's self-report of symptoms and objective clinical findings and observations during a physical exam. Additional disease discovery tools include lab test results, X-rays or digital scans, and genomic studies.

Do Not Resuscitate Form (DNR): An advance directive that is provided to health care professionals to authorize your loved one's wish of not being resuscitated if the heart stops or if your loved one stops breathing. The DNR is placed in one's medical health record or chart and is signed by a physician.

Documentation Plan: A backup plan to ensure that your documents can be located and found in a timely manner in the event the originals are lost or stolen.

Durable Power of Attorney for Health Care: A document giving legal authority to a designated person (i.e., caregiver) to make health care decisions on behalf of the loved one. It is also known as a health care proxy. This means that the designated person, or agent, may authorize or refuse medical treatment for the loved one. This power is activated by the loved one's physician but goes into effect only once the loved one is unable to make decisions for him- or herself.

Elder Care: Includes a range of services for the care and maintenance of the aged.

Elder Care Attorney: An attorney who specializes in the area of seniors. They have insight and experience with seniors and their unique needs. Common areas are estate planning, durable power of attorney for health care, wills, trusts, and Medicare and Medicaid.

Electronic Health Record (EHR): Patient-centered records that bring together content from multiple reliable and secure sources, such as from a lab, a hospital, an imaging center, emergency facilities, pharmacies, or treatment from other physicians.

Electronic Medical Record (EMR): Robust and secure software that allows only authorized providers to create, store, amend, and transmit patient medical records. The software, embedded inside the provider's tablet, also includes intelligence to the licensed clinician of your key data, such as food and drug allergies, current medications, and disease history.

Eligibility: An employee or his or her spouse, children, or domestic partner who meets requirements in a contract established by the employer and insurance company who pays for health insurance. Eligibility requirements may include the hours or years of employment or contract work.

Employee-Based Insurance Policy: Insurance provided by employer to the employee for coverage.

End of Life (EOL): Symptoms and body characteristics that indicate the body is near death. Often these symptoms offer comfort to caregivers, relieving them from fear and also helping other family members cope with the final stages of life.

Explanation of Benefits (EOB): A document produced by the health insurance company that explains services provided, amount billed to the insurance company, amount paid, and your balance due. An EOB is usually paid the day after funds are remitted to the provider so that you can compare the amount billed to you with the EOB's statement on what you owe.

Federal Trade Commission (FTC): An agency within the U.S. federal government that protects consumers. In this book, the FTC is mentioned as the agency that regulates funeral directors.

Financial Planner: A certified individual who helps people plan investments and make the best choices about investments or pensions.

Financial Power of Attorney: A document giving a designated person or persons the authority to make legal and financial decisions on behalf of the loved one. As the caregiver, it is important to know what authority you do and do not have with the power of attorney.

Funeral: A ceremony for someone who has died, usually held immediately before burial or cremation.

Funeral Director Meeting: A gathering of family members who meet with the funeral director to carry out the deceased person's wishes. Common topics include gathering legal documents, selecting a casket or urn, times of visiting hours and services, newspaper notices, and burial location.

Genetic Information Nondiscrimination Act (GINA): A law that prevents health plans from denying you coverage based on a genetic test that says you may carry the same gene for a specific disease in your family. For example, in caring for a parent with Alzheimer's disease, you may want to know if the disease is in your genes. A health plan that pays for the genomic test may not use your test results to underwrite your health coverage.

Group Insurance Policy: Insurance usually obtained through an employer, a professional or social organization, and a bank or credit agency.

Handheld Medical Devices: A small computer that can fit in one's hand. A cell phone, tablet, and smartphone are examples of handheld devices used in medicine.

Health Care Durable Power of Attorney: A legal document that designates an agent or proxy to make health care decisions if the patient is no longer able to make them. The surrogate person may function as the "attorney in fact" and make decisions, including cessation of treatment.

Health and Human Services (HHS): The federal agency that provides building blocks that Americans need to live healthy, successful lives.

Health Savings Account (HSA): Nontaxable savings accounts you create to help pay for health care costs. You, not your employer or insurance company, own the HSA. To be eligible for an HSA, you must combine your savings account with a high-deductible health plan.

High-Deductible Health Plan (HDHP): A high-deductible health plan lowers your monthly insurance fees, and it also raises the deductible amount, typically up to $5,000 to $10,000 per year, that you agree to pay out of pocket before the insurance kicks in. HDHPs are designed more for catastrophic health coverage than for preventive care. The more risk you accept on the front end, the lower your premiums. If you choose an HDHP plan, you also should consider tax savings by blending your HDHP with a health savings account. *See* Health Savings Account.

HIPAA: Health Insurance Portability and Accountability Act of 1996. HIPAA is a complex regulation that requires national standards for electronic health care transactions, code sets, national identifiers, and security. To protect confidentiality of personal health information, health care providers who bill electronically using HIPAA standards must adopt privacy and security requirements. If you feel your privacy has been breached, you can file a complaint with the provider or with the Office for Civil Rights.

Hospice: A special way of caring for people who have been diagnosed as terminally ill. Hospice care engages teams of clinicians, family members, clergy, and trained counselors who collectively address the medical, physical, social, emotional, and spiritual needs of the patient and the patient's family and caregiver.

Identity Theft: The taking of one's personal identification to assume that person's identity and to commit unlawful acts.

Individual Insurance Policy: An insurance policy purchased by an individual rather than offered by an employer.

Insurance Plan: A contractual agreement you make with an organization that you will pay a regular fee, and, in exchange, the plan will reimburse you for expenses as they are incurred. Your plan can reimburse the health care provider if you agree to let the provider file on your behalf. Commonly used insurance terms can be found at eHealthinsurance.com.

Joint Account: A bank account that has two equal owners or individuals who share access to the same account.

Letter of Testamentary: Sometimes called a letter of administration or representation. A document granted by a local court stating that you are the legal executor for a particular estate and that you have the ability to act as such.

Living Trust: A document giving a designated person, also known as a trustee, the authority to hold and distribute property and funds for the loved one once he or she is no longer capable of managing finances.

Living Will: An advance directive that describes and instructs how the loved one wants his or her end-of-life health care managed. This means that your loved ones decide in advance, while of sound mind and body, the kind of medical care they desire to receive or have withheld in the event they are unable to make their wishes known, such as the use of a ventilator, a feeding tube, or dialysis.

Long-Term Care: Includes medical and nonmedical care for people of any age who need help with daily living activities. Long-term care can be provided in the home, at an assisted living facility, or in a skilled nursing facility.

Long-Term Care Facility: Also called a skilled nursing facility. A place that provides medical and nonmedical care for people who are unable to perform basic activities of daily living, such as dressing or bathing, or for people who require rehabilitation services that exceed those that can be delivered in the home.

Low-Impact Movement: Using large-muscle groups in continuous rhythmic activity to decrease injuries. Low-impact exercises include walking, bicycling, swimming, dancing, yoga, Pilates, and balance exercises.

Medicaid: A joint federal and state program that helps with medical costs for individuals with limited resources. Medicaid programs vary from state to state.

Medical Billing Advocates: Organizations that will review your medical bill and help you dispute your bill. Typically, a medical billing advocate reviews complex hospital billing codes to identify obscure or confusing terms and help you resolve fees.

Medical Error: The definition of a medical error is a legal decision that involves negligence (failure to meet the standard of care) and preventable adverse events (failure to follow accepted practice).

Medical Tourism: Traveling to another state or another country to find a physician or hospital that specializes in treatment you may not be able to afford or find in the United States.

Medicare: A federal health insurance program for people who are over sixty-five years of age, certain younger people with disabilities, and people with end-stage renal disease who require dialysis and who are waiting for a kidney transplant.

Medication Management: The process of monitoring the medication of your loved one. The facilitation of safe and effective use of medicine (prescribed and over the counter) for your loved ones.

Memorial: A commemorative service honoring a person who is deceased. A memorial serves to preserve the memory of that person. Memorial services may take place within a day or two of death or can be delayed since the body is not present at the service.

Mobile Apps: Software designed to run on smartphones, mobile devices, or tablet computers. Apps are individual software units that have limited functions. The app may have links to more robust capabilities that you can use on your laptop or desktop computer.

Mortgage Life Insurance: Life insurance policies are incorporated into the mortgage payments and will pay off the mortgage on death.

Mortgage Statement: A statement from a financial institution that shows the mortgage principal and payments required.

National Academy of Elder Law Attorneys (NAELA): An association dedicated to servicing the needs of the aged population with education and advocacy. Provides a directory of elder care attorneys in the United States.

National Association of Unclaimed Property Administrators (NAUPA): The association of state unclaimed property programs with the responsibility of helping to reunite property owners with their unclaimed property.

Notice of Privacy Practices (NPP): Describes how a provider will use and disclose your protected health information for treatment, payment, or health care operations. Health care providers are required to post an NPP on websites or in plain view in the waiting room.

Obituary: A written announcement of death published in online and print newspapers that often includes a short biography, tribute, or short eulogy.

Office of Civil Rights: Agency within the U.S. Department of Health and Human Services with authority to enforce HIPAA Privacy and Security Rules.

Online Backup Storage: Remote backup. The storing of data off-site that is done regularly and tested.

Palliative Care: An approach to pain management offering relief of mental and physical pain without curing the disease. Palliative care is often sought for patients with a terminal illness.

Password: A string of characters to prove that you have the right to access information and the second part of the user authentication process. When combined with a unique user identifier, the password creates a mathematical equation, or algorithm, that says you are who you say you are.

Patient Portal: A secure 24-hour-per-day website that allows patients to access their health history, such as the name of your physician, your medications, immunization history, lab results, and much more.

Payable on Death: The owner of an account designates a beneficiary to receive all of the account assets immediately on death.

Personal Health Record (PHR): A paper or electronic summary of your personal health information for which you have control over the content, use, and security. Your PHR should, at a minimum, contain current medications, emergency contacts, severe allergies, and a brief overview of your medical history (e.g., diabetes mellitus type 2 since 2001).

Personal Representative: A person you legally appoint to make decisions on your behalf. For example, caregivers are frequently personal representatives for individuals who do not have the mental or physical capacity to make medical decisions. Personal representatives are treated with the same respect and authority as if they were the patient. Be sure you have a signed health care durable power of attorney.

Plan Accumulations: This is the total out-of-pocket expenses you paid to reach your deductible amount. Plan accumulations differ according to the health insurance plan you purchased.

Privacy Official: The person inside the practice, hospital, or health plan responsible for keeping your protected health information secure and private.

Procedure Codes: These are codes developed by the American Medical Association to identify services or procedures medically necessary to improve or stabilize your health. Procedures codes identify the service.

Protected Health Information (PHI): PHI is any demographic, clinical, or financial information that can be used to distinguish you from other individuals. This includes your past, present, or future (such as DNA tests) physical or mental health information or condition; health care you received; or past, present, or future payment provisions. If your information has been deidentified, or stripped of eighteen pieces of data, it is no longer PHI.

Reclaim: To take ownership of once again.

Remission: Slowing of a disease process or lessening of symptoms. A disease can be in remission for a few months or for a lifetime. In cancer treatment, remission means the patient is successfully responding to treatment. Complete remission may be considered cured.

Request Restrictions: A written request that you complete indicating that there is information in your medical chart that you do not wish disclosed to another person. For example, you agree to pay out of pocket for a service but do not want information about this procedure or treatment to be sent to your health plan.

Right to File a Complaint: If you believe that you or your loved one's privacy has been breached, you have a right to file a complaint with the provider or with the U.S. Department of Health and Human Services. The provider may not deny you with treatment or ask you to sign a waiver for treatment to keep you from filing a complaint.

Risk Management: The process of identifying, assessing, and prioritizing risks. It is the process of reducing risks due to certain types of events. Also known as a backup plan.

Savings Statement: A statement from a financial institution regarding a savings account balance.

Second Opinion: A visit to another physician you have not previously seen to get a different point of view or different approach to treatment. You may trust the first physician's assessment but still request a second opinion. Sometimes insurance companies require a second opinion.

Security: In electronic health records, security refers to measures put in place to ensure that the right information is accessed by the right person when needed. Security also means putting measures in place to keep unauthorized individuals, viruses, or malicious software from accessing your information.

Smartphone: A mobile phone with built-in applications and the ability to use the Internet.

Social Media: Interaction among friends, family, and coworkers of your loved one in which they can share, create, and exchange information over the Internet.

Summary of Charges: An overview of charges that the provider billed the insurance company. You should ask for claim details if the summary does not provide sufficient information.

Superbill: This is an itemized form that reflects the services provided by a licensed clinician. Information on your superbill is used to file a health care claim. Superbills are not uniform, but each superbill must contain four main parts: the name of provider and signature, the name of provider who referred you (if applicable), your patient information, and details in procedure and diagnostic codes.

Technology Plan: A layered process that preserves, protects, and manages the individual's "digital legacy."

Telemedicine: The exchange of medical information from one location to another via the use of electronic communication for the health and education of a patient.

Transfer of Assets: The process of moving one's assets to another account.

User ID: The unique combination of letters, numbers, or symbols that identify you from any other person attempting to access electronically stored information. When combined with a unique password, your user ID creates an algorithm that securely authenticates you.

Virtual Clinic: An optional location where a patient can participate in an interactive education and diagnosis from a physician via the computer rather than from home.

Virtual Office: A type of telemedicine where the patient can participate in video-conferencing with doctors through computers, tablets, and smartphones rather than a face-to-face visit with the physician.

Vital Signs: Your vital signs are signs of life. Typically, these include blood pulse rate, respiratory rate, body temperature, and blood pressure. Vital signs vary by age and may include pain level and the amount of oxygen in the lungs and bloodstream.

Voice-Over-Internet Protocol (VOIP): A technology where one can provide voice communications over the Internet.

Webcam: A video camera that streams images in real time to a computer or network. Caregivers may sometimes use a webcam to remotely monitor their loved ones.

Will: A document indicating how the loved one's assets and estate will be distributed among beneficiaries after the loved one's death.

Index